DREAMING OF STUTTERING FREEDOM

Speak with Confidence and Belief

RAMA SIVA

Thank you for purchasing this book. I congratulate you on embarking on a journey of freedom that will transform your life.

Here is a **SPECIAL GIFT** that will help you on your journey to stuttering freedom. Just go to this link below to get all the **bonus materials** that accompany this book.

www.thestutteringmind.net/bonus

For information contact Intrinsic Publishing.
Published by
Intrinsic Publishing
Intrinsic IT Ltd
10-12 Exchange Road, Stevenage SG1 1PZ
ISBN: 9781983097317

www.ramasiva.com
www.richthinking.net
www.thestutteringmind.com

Also by Rama Siva
Rich Thinking (Prequel to The Stuttering Mind Series)
The Rich Thinking Journal (available Winter 2018)
The Rich Shepherd (available Winter 2020)

The Stuttering Mind Series
Dreaming of Stuttering Freedom
Awareness of Stuttering Freedom (available Spring 2019)
Realising Stuttering Freedom (available Autumn 2019)
Experiencing Stuttering Freedom (available Spring 2020)

This book is dedicated to you.

Know that you are part of the One-mind which is both the actor and the spectator

.

Know that reality is much greater that you can possibly comprehend.

Know that the stuttering could be your greatest teacher, if you let it.

I am grateful to the many teachers who have helped me learn the truths.

I am grateful to be of service in sharing these with you.

Namaste

TABLE OF CONTENTS

Table of Contents..5

Foreword...7

The Extraordinary Mind 9

Day 67: The Birth...14

Day 68: The Return..18

Day 69: Princess..21

Day 70: Stuttering Redefined 24

Day 71: Pain Of Stuttering 28

Day 72: The Stuttering Triangle.................................32

Day 73: Stuttering Paradox......................................36

Day 74: Stuttering Voodoo 40

Day 75: The Truth 44

Day 76: The Brain Repairs Stuttering 49

Day 77: Three Months..56

Day 78: Ambushed 62

Day 79: Holding back..65

Day 80: The Fluency Trap 67

Day 81: Iceberg...70

Day 82: Classroom...72

Day 83: Proof Of Heaven 77

Day 84: Back To Earth...81

Day 85: Know Thyself 85

Day 86: What Do You Believe?....................................90

Day 87: You Are Not A Victim 94

Day 88: Dreams 98

Day 89: Habit 100

Day 90: Fears..102

Day 91: The Voice..104
Day 92: The Recovering Stutter 115
Day 93: Fluent or Non-Stutters 117
Day 94: Stuttering Paralysis 119
Day 95: Priceless...121
Day 96: The Power Within 123
Day 97: Hologram..126
Day 98: Manifesting Reality 129
Day 99: Matrix Reloaded 132
Epilogue 136
Awareness 141
One Last Thing..147
Facebook Group 148
Sources..149

FOREWORD

By John C. Harrison

This is the second in a remarkable series of books that Rama Siva is writing on the stuttering system, and it represents a new and effective way of understanding one of mankind's oldest mysteries.

We live at a time when we think nothing of building impossibly complex systems that do a better job at solving "unsolvable" problems. Space travel, exotic diseases, new and complex social systems -- nothing seems to defeat us anymore. Yet we continue to remain at a standstill when it comes to developing answers to one of mankind's most persistent puzzles.

What in the world is chronic stuttering really all about? And why, 5,000 years after the Old Testament first reported that Moses was "slow of tongue" in talking with God, have we still not been able to explain what drives chronic stuttering, and what we can do to solve it?

What is finally emerging is a new and evolving awareness that for all these years we've been trying to solve the wrong problem. We're not looking at a speech problem, per se. We're looking at a life system that involves not only a person's speech but the entire individual – how he thinks, how he perceives, and how he feels. It calls for us to take a giant step backward and look at a much bigger landscape than we've been surveying.

Rama Siva has a unique background that lends itself to this new perspective. Rama's roots into stuttering go back to his earliest years when as a very bright but very frightened young boy, he was "afraid to say boo to a goose." He would do everything possible not to have to express himself. He lived in a world of "self doubt, limiting beliefs and zero confidence." And as he was later to discover, he created the world that designed and maintained his stuttering.

This book is an account of Rama's unfolding analysis of his stuttering system and how he facilitated his transformation into a confident, creative and outspoken individual. By traveling with Rama on his voyage of self-discovery, and by looking carefully over his shoulder at how he went about disassembling the system that choked back his power, you will discover the unlimited horizons that lie within all of us...including you.

THE EXTRAORDINARY MIND

You are reading this because you are a parent of a child who stutters or in fact you are a person who stutters and are looking for answers. For over 25 years, my mum worried about how I would 'overcome' the stutter. She left this physical world in 2010 and this made me an angry young man. I was angry with the world for taking my mother so suddenly, angry with my father thinking why my mother and not him and angry with myself for not making my mother proud of me. In fact I was angry just because I was hurting. Even though I couldn't speak I always had a way with words. When I was 30, I wrote a letter to my parents telling them I will be better than all right. And now, as I write this book, I know this to be the case.

I was always a dreamer. I imagined a life without the stuttering companion. Since the age of 8, when I was labelled a stutterer and sent to speech therapy, I dreamt of a life free from inhibitions. At a young age, even though I stumbled over words and hesitated when speaking, I wasn't aware I was doing anything out of the ordinary. It didn't bother me. It was in the labelling of being a stutterer and the subsequent feelings of being different that made me self-conscious.

There was even a period of 2 weeks when I was mute, simply because since I couldn't speak properly, I decided I wouldn't speak. But I could speak, at least to myself out aloud when reading or talking to my cat. I was always perplexed, as to why I could speak properly to my cat and not to any human being. After many years of extensive thought, reading and contemplation I now know the answer. It was all in the stuttering mind.

You are in fact the greatest manifestation of the creation. You have unlimited capabilities, unbounded potential and extraordinary abilities, only limited by the stuttering mind. It was this mind, programmed and conditioned by external forces that led me to living an inhibited life. The life I led was one that was based on fear and the opinions of others. It meant not taking risks, not asking girls out, not demanding pay rises and not being the expression of life.

The stuttering was a crutch, an excuse not to live life. All through life, I sat on the sidelines. Never one to put my head above the parapet for fear of it being chopped off, I was too scared to say boo to a goose. If I had an opinion that was contradictory, I would keep quiet. Unknown to me, this way of living was slowly killing me. I had gone through life on the substitutes bench waiting to be picked, where in fact, it was I who had put myself there. Truth be told, the stutter was a manifestation of my personality. I can only speak about myself. All I know now, the beliefs I had, were not conducive to expressing myself. I had locked in the opinions of others, as truths, thus meaning I was living a life other than my own. My world was based on self-doubt, limiting beliefs and zero confidence.

After writing my first book, Rich Thinking, which is the prequel to the Stuttering Mind book series, the stuttering dissipated. I had assimilated the insights I had got from interviewing successful people and by going after my dreams this allowed my subconscious to let go of the fears and beliefs I had developed in childhood.

And so now, it my greatest wish that I can somehow help seventy million people to become free from the stuttering mindset. In this book series I will share my life experiences and how I am now free from the shackles of stuttering.

The D A R E principles are a 4 step process I coined in Rich Thinking.
- Dreaming - Without a dream where will you go?
- Awareness - Of your beliefs, emotions, feelings, thoughts, perceptions, environment, habits and actions
- Realising - You are the creator of your own life
- Experiencing - Make your dreams come true

Book 1, Dreaming of Stuttering Freedom, will show you the utmost importance of having a dream for your life and how this will help you to become free of the stuttering mind-set. By cultivating visons for your life in your mind's eye, through the power of your imagination you can not only become free from stuttering, but will be free to choose your experience of life. Life is a wonderful magical gift from the creator, of which you are a part of and it is for you to dream it into your experience.

As I wrote in Rich Thinking - 66 Days To Freedom:

'British writer James Allen states in As a Man Thinketh (1903): "Until thought is linked with purpose, there is no intelligent accomplishment. With the majority, the bark of thought is allowed to drift upon the ocean of life. Aimlessness is a vice, and such drifting must not continue for he who would steer clear of catastrophe and destruction. They who have no central purpose in their life fall an easy prey to petty worries, fears, troubles and self-pitying, all of which lead, just as surely as deliberately planned sins (though by a different route), to failure, unhappiness and loss, for weakness cannot persist in a power-evolving universe."'

You cannot be successful if you don't have a plan. You cannot be free from stuttering if you don't have a plan. This plan should be written down on paper. You need to have a vision, a roadmap to stuttering freedom, and only then will success be forthcoming. You need to develop unshakeable belief in your ability to create the life of your dreams. Anything is possible in this physical realm that we have manifested in. Everything exists with the word of God.

Book 2, Awareness of Stuttering Freedom will cover the importance of being aware of your beliefs, thoughts, emotions, feelings, perceptions, habits and actions. It is with your inner mind that your outer reality of your life and the stuttering is experienced. This second book will be published in Spring 2019.

Eric Edmeades shared in my book Rich Thinking:

"I have this idea that beliefs are a little bit like a living organism: they need food, and the food of beliefs is evidence." And the way in which a living organism keeps alive is by feeding. Edmeades explains, "Belief is like a little living organism and it's going to look around for food, and so if somebody believes that there's no opportunity, they will read about other people's ideas and they will respond with a 'Oh, look. Another idea that's gone.' Or if somebody else has a really nice car, or is really successful, then, the negative person will say that all the opportunities are gone. And that negativity will get stronger and stronger. But I look at this the other way around. I want to feed the beliefs in the right way. I want to feed the positive beliefs. I believe there are opportunities around every corner, and you know what, I see them all the time. It doesn't mean I have to pursue them, but I see them. I see them for what they are and I am able to make a decision as to whether I want to chase down a given opportunity."

As a person who stuttered for over 30 years, this had a profound impact on my life. What I know for sure, is that the beliefs I developed as a child are no longer needed as a 42 year old man. The stutter no longer serves me and there is no need for me to carry on stuttering.

Book 3, Realising Stuttering Freedom will cover aspects of creation. Have you ever wondered what was behind the Big Bang? How did we all come to live on planet Earth? The creator in his infinite wisdom created us with that creative spark in each and every one of us. We can either use this to create or destroy. For the creator it is just an experience. It is experiencing its creation through us. We are like actors on a giant stage called life. However, we are also the directors as well as the writers of our own lives. Have you ever considered you are on this planet called Earth that is spinning at a thousand miles an hour around the sun along with 8 other planets in perfect orbit? Can you see yourself from outer space walking or driving along and do you realise how amazingly lucky you are to be experiencing life on this playground? With our thoughts, beliefs, emotions, perceptions, feelings, habits and actions, we shape our world as we know it. Given that we are creators of our own reality, without a doubt we have the power within us to realise freedom from stuttering.

Believe it or not, the greatest scientist in the world, Albert Einstein said this so beautifully, "A human being is part of the whole called by us universe, a part limited in time and space. We experience ourselves, our thoughts and feelings as something separate from the rest. A kind of optical delusion of consciousness. This delusion is a kind of prison for us, restricting us to our personal desires and to affection for a few persons nearest to us. Our task must be to free ourselves from the prison by widening our circle of compassion to embrace all living creatures and the whole of nature in its beauty...We shall require a substantially new manner of thinking if mankind is to survive."

Book 4, Experiencing Stuttering Freedom will put all the pieces together. As we will establish, your current reality is based on your current thinking, which has been primarily created from your subconscious mind, based on years of programming picked up from childhood. This needs to be transformed so that you become the best version of yourself - now!

Achieving this takes desire to do so and you need to delve deep in your mind to make the changes in your life. Your subconscious mind needs to become aligned with your goals and your conscious mind, so they all start working together.

This book series is not for those who want an instant cure to stuttering. It has taken you years to get to where you are currently and granted there are some of you who will experience profound shifts while reading and doing the exercises; and will become free almost instantly. However for most of you, it will take time. Through the experiences of time you will no doubt be able to change the inner workings of your mind and start to have fun speaking. I now really enjoy taking to strangers in supermarkets. I enjoy smiling at people. It is amazing how a smile is contagious.

This book series is for those who want to explore the possibility of another way than that of traditional speech therapy treatments. I am not able to say that you will never stutter again, but what I know for sure that applying all these insights has freed me from the stuttering mindset.

You should also know that like anything in life that is worth getting, it takes hard work, determination, persistence and focus. Like in any walk of life, a mentor will usually give you a shortcut to success.

You can certainly use all the tools and techniques described in this book series, but if you find you are not making much headway then a mentor can certainly help you. Please do contact me at hellorama@thestutteringmind.com if I can be of help.

Acknowledgements

I would like to thank Dr Christian Kell, Dr Eben Alexander, Robert Schwartz and Karen Newell for their time in being interviewed for this book.

I would like to thank my wife, son and my parents for their support in always pursuing my dreams.

Thank you to all my mentors, some of whom I have met in person and others I have found in the numerous books I have read in my quest for stuttering freedom.

DAY 67: THE BIRTH

It happened. I was 8 years old and in school reading out aloud. Reading books about pirates, lost treasure and adventure was my favourite past time. I would spend hours getting lost in that world and would bring those pirates and dragons to life.

"The ppppirates bbbboarded tttthheee sssssshiiip," I stuttered as I read aloud one afternoon. I continued, "Sssstop shouted the ccccaptain." This was the first time I recall stuttering. It wasn't something that I was worried about, but that was the moment, I now recall, as the time I was sent direct to the speech therapy jail.

I call it jail as, in that second, my teachers labelled me a person who was different and that label would be superglued to my psyche for over 30 years.

Self-doubt had slowly but surely crept into my mind. I didn't know what the word meant but that would result in a life time of holding back and not participating in the game of life.

A part of me was afraid of speaking. I could read out aloud, perfectly well when alone, however when I was in front of other people, my subconscious would make it my reality that I stuttered. I had developed self-doubt in my ability to speak and this manifested itself as hesitations, repetitions, adding filer words such as 'humm' or 'ah' which led to blocking and finally being labelled as a stutterer. That part of me wasn't comfortable expressing itself. It was scared. I felt as if a snake had wrapped itself around my throat and chest areas preventing me from speaking. It was fearful of being judged, made fun of and laughed at. That part of me was still a child that needed love and protection. The inner child within all of us needs to be shown we are truly part of the Divine and there is nothing to be fearful of.

Life, as I now realise, is a drama, something like "Eastenders," a British TV series, where every day you have a chance to really live with joy and happiness; or in the case of "Eastenders" shout and bitch about life. From the first moment I watched "The Matrix" in 1999, it blew my mind away. The special effects and mind bending plot made cinema history. It was only later on in life, that I thought what if there was an underlying message to the Matrix? Is it possible that reality isn't what we think it is? Now quantum physicists are saying there is nothing solid about the universe. We are, in effect, living in a hologram. There will be more about the Matrix in Book 3 of The Stuttering Mind.

When Buddha said 'Life is suffering,' he saw the physical aspects of suffering in the hunger of the poor. As a person who stutters, the suffering was in my mind. Years of sitting on the sideline, due to holding back, meant I was in the jail of the self-imposed limitations.

However I had a vision, it was just a passing conversation with Matthew, while I was working at the Forensic Science Service in London. He commented, "In the basement of 10 Downing Street, there is a computer suite." This conversation took place in October 1998. Two years later I would attend an interview at the Prime Minister's Office.

I stuttered, "I aaaammmm hhhhere to attend a job interview," as I showed my interview letter and passport to the policeman at the gates of No10.

I knocked on the famous black door and entered. The words, "First Lord Of The Treasury" would be forever etched into my memory. Stepping in through that door, I marvelled at the grandeur of the lobby area. The chandeliers that hung from the ceiling made it even more impressive. I left my mobile phone in a secure cabinet and was escorted to the waiting area. The heating was on and the room was lovely and warm. I tried to remain calm as I was reading through some notes I had made in preparation for my interview. I had always found interviews to be one of my most stressful situations and realised that preparation was the key to success. I was well qualified for the job so I knew I could easily do it. I had studied, each evening for four hours a day to pass my Microsoft IT exams, within six months. Now, I just had to control my speech for the next hour to land my dream job.

Finally, one of the staff came and escorted me up to one of the state rooms. Known as the Pillared Room, its giant white pillars were the main feature. Priceless paintings hung on the wall. I looked around marvelling at the décor of the room. I was lucky my interview was being held there. In the far corner, by the window, facing Horse Guard's Parade sat three people. Philip, Wendell and Rosie. I was nervous as hell. I wanted this job. Just walking in and feeling the sense of history made me full of joy and enthusiasm. I loved being there. I opened my mouth and spoke. Yes, I stuttered here and there, but I did well in the interview. I soaked in the atmosphere and history of the place before leaving No10. I didn't know if I would return.

What do Moses, Aristotle, Charles Darwin, King George, Julia Roberts, Nicole Kidman and Ed Sheeran all have in common? They all had a stutter. Ever since I was a teenager I always wondered and asked my parents why I stuttered and what did I do to deserve this pain. That was over 30 years ago. I know now the answer. I never ever thought I would actually be grateful for having a stutter. In all those years I suffered from heartache, disappointment, shame, fear and loneliness. These aren't the only words I could use; the list would fill up this chapter so I will stop with the five I have written so far.

Having a stutter profoundly affected the way I viewed the world. This meant not having close friends, socializing or snogging girls behind the bike shed. My teenage years were filled with idly day dreaming my life away. I flunked out of school. I barely got into college. I was depressed and didn't know it. I could see no light at the end of the tunnel. It was my belief, I would stutter, until the end of my days. The stutter completely and utterly ruled my life. I would wake up each morning, remembering I stuttered and so the day went. I went for job interviews at local supermarkets and was politely rejected. There was a point, in my job searching process that I ticked the disability box and wrote I had a stutter. But to no avail. I was still unable to find a permanent job. I had a stutter and was poor financially. Not a great combination when it came to dating.

Thankfully at the age of 18, I attended a two week intensive speech therapy course at my local hospital, before I started college. Otherwise I might have given up on life. School was hell. I had friends at school but never actually felt part of the school. I didn't enjoy life at school. Many people say that their school years were the best, well for me they were the worst. Kids can be so cruel. I was glad to have left my school years behind.

The first day at Oaklands College was filled with nerves. I sat quietly at the back of the class and in walked a middle aged balding gentleman. He introduced himself as "C C C o o l l i i i n." He stuttered more than I did. He was to be my form tutor for the next nine months. I was religiously practicing speaking out aloud repeating, "The goldfish and the gerbil are said to make very good pets" story, which I listened to on the car tape player as I drove to college every day. This exercise helped me to maintain what little control and confidence I had in my ability to speak. I don't know if it was fate or coincidence, but having Colin as my teacher helped me settle in. I did well that year in college and got a place at university. I never thanked Colin for being a teacher in spite of having a stutter. I can't imagine the courage he needed to have, teaching especially to rowdy teenagers.

In college, I met a girl who was my friend. Her name was Donna. Since I failed my A- levels I had to go to a college in Welwyn Garden City to enter university the following year. All the students on the Business and Computing foundation course had failed their exams too. So they obviously all had issues in their lives. As a stutterer, I thought I was the only one with a problem. Donna was a single mum. She was kind to me and we were good friends along with Andy P.

Spending time with Andy Yo, Joseph who wanted to be called James, Asif, Vishal and another friend whose real name was James, my time at the college was enjoyable. Playing snooker with Andy Yo and Vishal was a weekly hobby. I enjoyed their company. However I was still reserved. I somehow found it easier to talk to Donna. I told her about the stutter and how I had been on a speech therapy course before coming to college. It was interesting for me to note that I had a friend despite the stutter. I had always imagined myself as being lonely forever and looking on with envy as the world went by. I was sad to find out that Donna had dropped out of college after Christmas. I got on with the other lads but I had lost a friend. Looking back I have always found it easier to converse with girls than boys. I felt more at ease, however when it came to girlfriends it was another story. It was like I had mental block that stopped me from taking a risk and sharing my true feelings.

In every class, there is a class clown, and we had a few at Oaklands College. In the wisdom of the class clown, one of them looked through Colin's briefcase and got a copy of an upcoming test paper. Needless to say, they all did really well in that particular exam. Colin was really pleased, thinking that his teaching had converted a bunch of failures to Oxford scholars. However, in the next exams the class clowns got their usual grades.

Buying a train ticket, when my car was out of action, was the highlight of my stuttering life during my college year. In the end I resorted to writing the destination on a piece of paper and showing it to the ticket vendor at the counter. Despite being on a two week speech therapy course I still hadn't cracked the stuttering nut. I would have to wait 23 years to have freedom from the stuttering mind as I write this book series.

Thought for the Day: "We are changed by what we do, not by what we think about, or read about, but by what we actually do." Winston Churchill

Talking Point: Recall the first time you became aware that you spoke differently. Were you with your family or friends? Or were you in school? What do you remember about that day?

Exercise: Close your eyes and try to relax. Breathe in deeply 3 times. Try to imagine you are back in that situation. How old are you? What can you see around you? What are you feelings in that moment? Do you have a sense of panic? Are you nervous? Or are you so excited that the words just seem to trip up as you speak. Now write all this down on paper.

DAY 68: THE RETURN

Entering university was scary. I had left home for the first time and was living in halls. There I met a couple of girls. One was Claire and the other was Alex. They were both friendly and outgoing which made me feel at ease. But I was still the shy boy with nothing much to say. This was first time I had to cook for myself, so frozen chicken kiev became a favourite of mine as it was quick and easy to bake in the oven. I had that along with pasta, pretty much every day.

The stutter had come back with a vengeance. Despite practicing speaking out aloud in the car to the goldfish and gerbil story I was struggling. I didn't have a word for it back then, but I now know it as holding back. When push came to shove I would speak. I would stutter quite a bit, but what was happening in University was I would avoid situations and people. I would stay in my room and not socialize with the rest of guys on my floor. Occasionally, I would venture out, but the majority of the time, I would be in my room. I had a huge life size poster of Cindy Crawford that hung on the wall by the door. And another of a red Ferrari that was by my bed. I still dream of meeting Cindy Crawford and driving a Ferrari. I think, I will get the Ferrari.

In my first days at University I met the most gorgeous petite girl called Sam. She was in all of my classes. She had the most beautiful eyes I had ever seen. She was mesmerizing. I was in love. I remember one day in lectures she was sat behind me with one of her friends. She was looking at me and I was looking at her. She waved to me. I smiled. I was on cloud nine for the rest of the day.

But I had a stutter that ruled my life which meant all the confidence I had was knocked out of me. I had never had a girlfriend, let alone a close friend who was a girl, apart from Donna. In school I had crushes on girls but was petrified of talking to them. Girls to me were like from another world, and so they remained an enigma.

Being of Sri Lankan Tamil descent meant I stood out in my school in the not so leafy suburbs of Hertfordshire, and having a stutter to boot meant I was like a clown at a wake. I would say, I am good looking but the experiences or rather the non-experiences with girls, made me see myself as ugly and unworthy of love. The fear of having braces for my teeth meant I looked like bugs bunny during my teenage years.

In my twenties I would have braces, but would still be girlfriendless. This belief would remain with me until I got married. Ever since Miss World and Miss Universe were shown on TV, it was my dream to marry a girl from Colombia or Venezuela. Looks like dreams do come true. I think I also saw Donald Trump make his first TV appearance in a swimsuit. Scary thought.

My first year of university wasn't a good experience. I was living away from home in university halls. Sure, I had some friends, but they were more like acquaintances. I felt so alone in a place full of students. I didn't drink alcohol and didn't particularly enjoy drinking beer as to me it tasted of piss. Well, I don't know what piss tastes like, but I imagine it being pretty similar to beer. I joined a couple of clubs but due to the stutter I wouldn't speak to anyone. I just didn't want them to find out my secret. The stutter limited my ability to make friends and so I didn't really have any.

Sam and I did a group assignment together, but I had no game. I just couldn't imagine why she would possibly be interested me. I became love sick and depressed. And once again I would wile away wasting my time. However, I managed to pass the exams to get through to the next year.

My second year wasn't getting any better. The first year crush on a girl came and went, and so another girl walked across my radar. I saw her from afar. It was like ground hog day. Her name was Sita. There was another girl that looked quite like her. One day Sita would have long hair and the next she would appear with short hair. I then realised she was a twin when I saw the two girls together.

It took me about two months to get up the courage just to say hi. I had seen Sita a number of times over the previous months at University. Despite the stutter I finally went over and introduced myself to her. The situation went well. She didn't laugh or slap me. I was absolutely terrified of speaking to her. I felt really proud that I spoke to her and introduced myself. It was a big first step.

Over the next few months I would see her and say "hi". However, I had no game. I was still the shy boy who didn't know how to converse with someone who I found attractive. I was lost in my world of self-doubt and fear. There was one evening, when I really wanted to talk to her. So I went up and said "hi". She said she was busy and had to go. In my mind, I felt rejected so left feeling desolate. I couldn't see that she was really busy and wanted to finish her coursework. All I could see and feel, was the feeling of rejection and heartache, that the girl I was interested in, didn't want to know me. So that was the end of Sita. In that moment my heart was broken and there was no return.

While love sick and depressed about my life I went to see a psychologist at my university. Interestingly, I saw another girl who I shared some of my classes with. It's strange, one thinks that you are the only person in the world, that has problems, so it was comforting to see another person, who I had known also seeing a psychologist. After having four sessions with her, the psychologist made me so mad that I thought to myself 'I am going to show you and make something of my life.' So I never returned.

While in the second year, I met a good friend who was from Germany. Oliver was on an exchange year and we had some economics classes together. One day Oliver and I were studying at a desk in the library, and Sita came and sat down next to me. We said "hi", and that's about it. I had no conversation skills. I was lost in the stuttering mind. That year I did really well in my exams. I guess going to see the psychologist helped me.

I was developing socially. Bambi, Jenny, Lorna and Nila were my closet friends in my final year at University. We had studied statistics together over the previous two years and enjoyed each other's company. I was still the reserved quiet one.

Thought for the Day: Part of me suspects I'm a loser, and part of me thinks I'm God Almighty. - John Lennon

Talking point: Recall any situation where you are able to speak with someone without worrying about the stutter. Was the stutter less pronounced? And recall in what situations the stutter took a life of its own. Can you now see that the stuttering was dependent on your comfort level?

Exercise: Once again close your eyes and relax. Try to imagine all the situations and people where you are completely at ease speaking. It doesn't matter if you stumble. There is a difference between stumbling over words and stuttering. Everyone stumbles over words from time to time. It is when you attach meaning to the stumbling that creates the problem of uncontrolled stuttering. Write down the complete list of situations and people where your speech didn't bother you. On a scale of 1 to 10, mark down where 10 was where your speech was great and you felt really good about yourself, and where 1 was the speech was acceptable and it didn't overly bother you that you stumbled quite a bit when speaking.

DAY 69: PRINCESS

My world changed when I met a beautiful and vivacious girl who was full of life and laugher. Zena was from Cyprus, and had a similar background to me, but in reverse. She had left the United Kingdom when she was 12 and returned when she was 18. I had spent most of my life abroad up until the age of 12. We got on really well and I felt comfortable in her presence. We studied together. She inspired me to study well and do well in my exams. We shared two economics classes a week so I would look forward to seeing her. Even though I would stutter when I was with her it didn't seem to matter. I fell in love with her. But I was too scared to do anything about it. The stutter was still ruling my life.

In the first two years at University I was pretty much depressed all of the time. I was alone and felt lonely in a university full of people. I felt so disconnected from everyone. I felt invisible. In the final year I felt I was somebody. I actually called people on the telephone and spoke to them.

All through my life I would ask myself, why do I stutter and thought it was a curse. All my friends could speak. Everyone I met could speak. I was the only person who couldn't string two words coherently together. There must be something wrong with me. I would have this thought repeating over and over in my mind. Why me? Why me? Why me? I hate my stutter. I hate my life. I want to die.

What changed for me was meeting Zena. For the first time in my life, I had a good friend who would telephone me. I could see that despite having a stutter I had a friend. I never had anyone telephone and want to talk to me. There was light at the end of the tunnel.

Back to the why me question. I now know the answer. It was to experience life as a stutterer, to feel the shame, feel the heartache, feel the loneliness and to come through it. Sadly, there are some who give up.

It was only in 2018, I came across the story of a young man who took his own life. Dominic Barker was a highly educated university graduate who had a stutter and struggled to find a job. This struggle would lead him to commit suicide. It was heart breaking for me to read this and this in turn has spurred me on to share my story to give hope to other stutterers who can't see a light at the end of the tunnel.

A friend of mine, shared his painful stuttering story of his marriage breaking up, when his wife threw him out of the family home, as she found him stuttering away to his youngest son while he reading a bed time story. Another friend shared his story of his arranged marriage not going through as the prospective parents in law found out he had a stutter. And, another friend shared his story of getting ready to end it all by taking 6 paracetamol tablets, but heard a voice telling him to google speech therapy.

There are many stutterers who have been on various speech therapy programs but to no avail. There are others who are addicted to different programs that essentially teach the same concepts. The search needs to begin on the inside and I humbly share my story with you.

In my own quest for freedom I have read and thought extensively as to, why me? How can any speech therapist know what a stutterer is going through unless they have had a stutter for any period of time? Now I can honestly say I am grateful to the stutter. After all, God chose Moses to reveal himself as "I am that, I am." And Moses had a speech impediment. Having a stutter has led me to an introspection of what is real and what isn't. I am not the body. I am the spirit inside the body. Our bodies are the temples of our spirits.

Quoting from the scriptures:

"Do you not know that your body is a temple of the Holy Spirit, who is in you, whom you have received from God? You are not your own; you were bought at a price. Therefore honor God with your body," (1 Cor. 6:19-20).

Jesus answered the unbelievers, "Is it not written in your law, 'I said, "You are gods"'? If He called them gods, to whom the word of God came (and the Scripture cannot be broken), do you say of Him whom the Father sanctified and sent into the world, 'You are blaspheming,' because I said, 'I am the Son of God'? If I do not do the works of My Father, do not believe Me; but if I do, though you do not believe Me, believe the works, that you may know and believe[d] that the Father is in Me, and I in Him." (John 10:34-38)

As we know the body is the temple, then they way to God is through the part of you that is God.

Jesus explained, "I am the way and the truth and the life. No one comes to the Father except through me. If you really know me, you will know my Father as well. From now on, you do know him and have seen him."

Philip said to Him, "Lord, show us the Father, and it is sufficient for us."

Jesus said to him, "Have I been with you so long, and yet you have not known Me, Philip? He who has seen Me has seen the Father; so how can you say, 'Show us the Father'? Do you not believe that I am in the Father, and the Father in Me? The words that I speak to you I do not speak on My own *authority*; but the Father who dwells in Me does the works. Believe Me that I *am* in the Father and the Father in Me, or else believe Me for the sake of the works themselves. (John 14:6-11)

Ever since a young age I never actually felt part of this world. I have always felt I was looking on from the outside in. I felt separate and alone. Writing this book has made me even more spiritually aware. The insights I gained from interviewing and then writing my first book, has been liberating. I have realised that we are all part of the 'One'. We never actually separated from God. The spirit that is in each one of us is the same. Just like a drop of water is part of the ocean, you are actually part of the universe. Once you can fathom the greatness and the magic of life then you will be free from the fear of not being good enough, the fear of unworthiness and be the vessel for the creator to experience life. You are perfect just the way you are. You don't have to change a thing. Just realise the inherent greatness within you.

Thought for the Day: Being deeply loved by someone gives you strength, while loving someone deeply gives you courage. Lao Tzu

Talking point: Jesus said, "You are Gods." Is it possible he has told us life's secret?

Exercise: If you are a Christian, start reading 9 verses of the Bible aloud every day. If you are not a believer, then read a chapter from Rich Thinking aloud every day.

DAY 70: STUTTERING REDEFINED

To stammer or to stutter, that is the question? Well it's the same. Stammer is normally used in the United Kingdom and stutter is the term used in the United States. Stuttering is a worldwide issue; it affects the rich and poor alike; affects men 4 times as many as women; and about one percent of the world's population which is about 70 million people.

Wikipedia defines, "Stuttering, also known as stammering, is a speech disorder in which the flow of speech is disrupted by involuntary repetitions and prolongations of sounds, syllables, words or phrases as well as involuntary silent pauses or blocks in which the person who stutters is unable to produce sounds. The term stuttering is most commonly associated with involuntary sound repetition, but it also encompasses the abnormal hesitation or pausing before speech, referred to by people who stutter as blocks, and the prolongation of certain sounds, usually vowels or semivowels."

Traditional therapies did not work for me. I had tried prolongation speech, easy onset, and even a headset to stop me hearing my own voice. I wanted to be beyond techniques and so my quest for freedom began. I knew that people such as former US Vice President Joe Biden stuttered until his 30s and over the years stopped, so there had to be a way for me to become free.

Stuttering freedom means to be able to express oneself without self-doubt and without holding back. To stumble over a sound or word is immaterial if there is no fear attached. If the seed of doubt is watered, then the fear will grow to an oak tree. If however, the roots are examined and weeded out, freedom beckons. How can you be fearful of yourself? There is only one universe, one song. All the great sages, teachers and mystics have passed on the message that we are all one. The illusion of separation is just that, an illusion. It is not what is appears to be. And once you work on the beliefs that are holding you back, the stutter will dissipate.

Stuttering for me is the unconscious pattern of hesitation and holding back when speaking. It's the repetition of sounds, words, or blocking coupled with facial distortions in the attempt to get a word out when speaking which developed into a lifetime fear of speaking as I didn't want to stutter and be laughed at. I was terrified in class. I didn't want to stand out and the stutter made me stand out. It was as if the inner being wanted me to stand out and be counted and not just blend in like I consciously wanted to. The mere repetitions of sounds or words doesn't constitute stuttering. If so Prime Minister Teresa May is a stutterer along with Mark Zuckerberg. Under pressure, everyone stumbles or stutters. That doesn't mean he or she is a stutterer.

Stuttering is such a broad term. There are many stutterers who live their lives in bliss irrespective of the stutter. It hasn't caused them to become a shrinking violet. However, there are many more stutterers who are greatly affected by the effects of stuttering. This may affect their choice of job, partner and even their mental health. Confidence, low self-esteem, social anxiety are effects of stuttering or is it the other way round?

I first met John Harrison, who was the former associate director of the National Stuttering Association in 2003 at a neurosematitics for stuttering workshop in London. He told me something that struck me, "Double your volume and half your speed when speaking." And yes, it's true I had more control over my speech when I was speaking slower and with the voice much louder than I was used to. However, there was no long lasting breakthrough. While on the workshop I met loads of other stutterers whose speech was worse than mine. Their stuttering minds weren't comfortable speaking with other stutterers, where as I was perfectly at ease.

There were people on the workshop who had severe blocking and struggles when speaking and there were others who seemed to be pretty fluent. However, since they were at that workshop, stuttering was still an issue in their lives.

In his book Redefining Stuttering, John Harrison proposes that the word stuttering is given up except in the broadest of discussions. In its place he suggests five different terms that describes perfectly the situation in which the disfluency occurs.

Pathological disfluency is defined as disfluencies related to primary pathology such as cerebral insult or intellectual deficit.

Developmental disfluency surfaces when a young child struggles to master the intricacies of speech. Harrison says." this is a developmental model all its own which is separate and distinct from the developmental model of adult blocking behaviour. Developmental disfluency often disappears on its own as the child matures. It is also highly receptive to therapeutic intervention, so much so that when treated early enough, most children attain normal speech without any need to exercise controls."

Harrison coined the term 'bobulating', to mean when someone has temporary disfluency when under stress. I know from personal experience that former UK Prime Minister Tony Blair 'bobulated'. No one labelled him a stutterer! Every human being bobulates to some degree. Harrison explains, "However, this is usually not a chronic problem, and even if it were, the person is generally unaware of his behaviour and is, therefore, unlikely to have negative feelings toward it."

The word blocking is used when describing the classic struggling and choking speech block that someone has when he has obstructed his airflow and constricted his muscles. This strategy has been developed by the subconscious mind to protect the speaker from unpleasant experiences. Harrison suggests, "that the person is blocking something from his awareness such uncomfortable emotions or self-perceptions."

Finally the fifth type of disfluency is called stalling, where Harrison describes it, "as when the person repeats and word or syllable because he has a fear that he will block on the following word or syllable." Harrison explains this strategy as when the speaker is trying to buy time until he is ready to say the dreaded word.

These five words perfectly encompasses all the scenarios of the stutter in his or her stuttering world. I was a staller and blocker. Now I "bobulate" from time to time. The words don't have any meaning. I refuse to be tattooed.

I defined goals that were conducive to motivating a person that is no longer afraid of speaking. For instance, one of my goals was to actually enjoy having conversations with people. To really get to know the individual as a person; to listen to what they say instead of being so worried about myself and the stutter. I found that the greatest conversation can be had when you are really listening to someone without any of the mental chatter. I did that when I interviewed so many famous people and it was so fascinating to see how they all overcame self-doubts. For someone who stuttered I thought I had the monopoly of doubts, but it became apparent that nearly everyone faced adversity. And, it is in the how you pick yourself up and get up off the canvas that determines if you will either make the breakthrough or give up.

Life is meaningless. It is you that gives it meaning. The creator gave you, life. You are the writer, director of and actor in of your own life. It is with your thoughts, beliefs, perceptions, emotions, feelings, habits and actions that you create your reality. It is you that gives meaning to events. When I stuttered while reading out aloud, I gave the stutter a meaning. It was something that I didn't want. By attaching a feeling that it was something bad and not to be repeated this meant my subconscious took it to mean that stuttering was bad. Over time, this grew to a fear of stuttering and then a fear of speaking.

Thought for the Day: "Don't treat it (stuttering) as an issue-work through it and get the treatment that you want to get, but don't ever treat it as an issue, don't see it as a plight on your life, and carry on pushing forward." Ed Sheeran

Talking point: Have you ever thought why you don't stutter every single time you speak? Have you ever examined what situations you are mostly 'fluent' and don't block or stutter?

Exercise: Write down in detail the situations where you stutter uncontrollably. Try to describe in as much detail as possible what the situation entailed. Who were you talking with? What was the subject matter? Were you trying to impress somebody?

Write down in detail the situations where you are mostly 'fluent'? Are you relaxed, comfortable and enjoying the time. Do you feel the need to speak or does the conversation flow naturally?

DAY 71: PAIN OF STUTTERING

I t was my good friend Entrepreneur, Chris Payne, who shared with me the story of the dog and the nail in my book Rich Thinking.

Payne explained why a lot of people fail when it comes to taking action with this anecdote, "A young man moves in to a new area and he goes out for a walk one evening. He walks around the block and he comes across a house set back from the road. There's a dog on the porch, and it's howling. Behind the dog is an old man who is gently rocking in a rocking chair."

"The young man carries on walking round the block, and as he comes around the block, the dog is still howling on the porch.''

"The young man walks down the path of the house, goes up to the old man and asks: 'Why is your dog howling?'''

"The old man pauses in his rocking chair and says: 'Well, it's probable that the dog is sitting on a nail.'''

"The young man says: 'So why doesn't the dog get off the nail?'''

"And the old man says: 'The nail probably doesn't hurt enough.'''

"In other words, you are not going to really make any money unless you have a valid reason to do so. And often, it's pain that's the most powerful motivator. When you are in pain with where you are, you act. You know, we have to have a motivator, because otherwise we put off tomorrow what we could do today and everyday becomes: 'I'll do that tomorrow.' And little is achieved."

Payne goes on to say "Mark Anastasi teaches this: in life, you are either moving towards pleasure or away from pain. So, some people are very excited about creating a six-figure income. But how many people put the energy into establishing how things work? Or into refocusing their personal priorities and changing the direction of their careers? Not that many at all."

That story had such a profound effect on my life. In my case it's perfectly true – the pain of stuttering wasn't big enough. People move towards pleasure and away from pain. That is part of being human. And being human is to experience life, take risks and live and having a stutter meant I wasn't living.

As a person who stuttered, I was in my comfort zone. The stutter wasn't that bad, my life wasn't that bad, really. I hadn't actually committed suicide. Sure, I wanted more from my life than hating the weekends, as I had no friends and nothing to do. The pain wasn't big enough.

The brain is there to protect you and do the least amount of work, so in this case, it did nothing. If I didn't go out, I wouldn't stutter. If I didn't do anything, I didn't stutter. I was lost in my own mind of comfort. Why was that? I was comfortable living with my loving parents, wasn't threatened by them and there was nothing that really pushed me to get out there.

And yet, I craved human company. I wanted to go out and meet girls, and yet I couldn't. I was still trapped in my mind of fear and self-doubt. And that remained with me for a very, very long time.

The shame, embarrassment, self-depreciation, fear, anxiety, nervousness, loneliness, depression, self-conscious, panic, anger, rejection, feeling of worthless and feeling of no one is going to love me meant a life time of sitting on the sidelines of life. I was too scared of living, so I was in effect dying.

It was 2009. I was working for the UK Foreign Office travelling the world. I was living my dream life. But there was a part of me that wasn't happy. Years earlier in university, I had met a girl. She had an impact on my life. University life wasn't much fun as a stutterer. I was lost in my own world of self-doubt and depression. We were good friends and she inspired me to study well. I fell in love with her laugh and personality. She was pretty hot too! And yet, despite being comfortable around her and not really worried about the stutter, I just couldn't see why she would be interested in me. The self-doubt has grown to become a monster that ruled my life. The pain of stuttering had just been tipped over the scales and I started to fight back at the 120 pound gorilla.

So let's begin...Are you interested in or committed to the idea of being free from the stutter? There is a difference: If you are interested you will just do enough to get by. I was like that for 16 years. If you are interested you will not wake up at 6am to read books and develop yourself. If you are interested you will attend speech therapy courses and stick in that comfort zone forever. If, however, you are committed to the process, you will do whatever it takes to be free from the stutter. If you are committed, you will increase your knowledge and skills so that you can speak with confidence and eloquence. If you are committed, you will transform your beliefs so that you are free to be the best version of yourself.

Grab an A4 sheet of paper and answer the following if you are committed to being free:

What is your reality of life as a stutterer? Write it down in as much detail as possible.

What do you do? Are you in a job that truly inspires you and that you are passionate about? Or if you didn't stutter you would be in a completely different career. What is stopping you? Really?

How does your stuttering manifest? Write it down

Are you actually comfortable having a stutter? Really? What would you do to change this?

What benefit does stuttering have for you?

Go to www.thestutteringmind.com/exercises to get all the worksheets that will help you in the quest to freedom.

If you would like a free 30 minute Skype consultation upon completion of these worksheets, please do contact me at hellorama@thestutteringmind.com

I had a dream of being an author and a speaker, and it was in August 2017 that I was interviewed on BBC radio in the United Kingdom. I was driving home listening to the repeat broadcast with my wife and son. It brought tears of joy and relief. It was a cathartic moment. My school life was hell. My college life was remarkably enjoyable thanks to a teacher who stuttered. My university life was depressing. I had built up the self-imposed limitations in my mind such that I wasn't able to live. A lifetime later, I would realise that the limitations were of my own making. Granted, there were external factors which contributed to how I was, but it was my reactions to these factors that led me to living or rather not living.

I was 41 years old and had stuttered all my life. Unfortunately, I had kept this stuttering habit for all this time, despite attending different speech therapy courses. I was addicted to speech therapy courses. I would come off a course flying high, and then would crash and burn. This course of events would be repeated over many years. Until I had enough! The pain of stuttering was finally big enough. I had a son and didn't want the same life experience for him. I had to reinvent myself.

In the process of interviewing 20 entrepreneurs including Allon Khakshouri, the former manager of Novak Djokovic, I had unconsciously released all the limitations that I had placed on myself. All these years, I had wanted so much to be able to speak without stuttering and despite the best of efforts and willpower I would not make a breakthrough of more than a few weeks. It was only after listening to the interviews that it was apparent I no longer stuttered or needed to stutter. There was no longer an excuse for me to carry on stuttering.

The dream of being an author and speaker was far greater than the need to stutter. There are many theories of stuttering as to hereditary or genetic nature. It may be true that both my cousin and his son also suffered from this predicament. However for me, thinking that, does not serve me any purpose.

Julia Roberts, Nicole Kidman, Emily Blunt and Ed Sheeran to just name 4 people have overcome stuttering. They have not let their limitation of stuttering stop them becoming very successful in their careers. This shows to me that it is actually possible in the realms to break free from the stuttering jail.

When I was 11 years old I wrote a prize winning essay about the solar system. If I didn't have a fear of speaking I would have read out my speech in front of the school. Alas, my fear of stuttering prevented me from living that experience. And to this day, I still remember that essay... and the regret of not facing the fear of speaking in front of my class.

Thought for the Day: "I remember a long time ago my Grandpa told me: 'Don't ever let anybody tell you that you can't do anything because you stutter." Darren Sproles

Talking point: What was your worst and best experience of speaking?

Exercise: Answer the questions that were posed and send an email to hellorama@thestutteringmind.com for a free skype consultation.

DAY 72: THE STUTTERING TRIANGLE

O ur experience of life is composed of 3 parts: The Body, the Mind and the Spirit. The physical aspect of our incarnation on this planet is the body. From the very moment of birth, it is said that we begin to forget our connection to the Spirit. Who is it that sees through the eyes? Who is it that listens through the ears? As a child I remember looking at the mirror as I aged. When I was 18, I wondered who was stuttering? Is it the 8 year old child or the 18 year old man? Who is afraid of expressing himself? As a 42 year old man I now realise I am the spirit who resides in this human body as it ages and experiences all the suffering. I am no longer afraid of expressing myself. I realise I am part of the creator and the experience. I am here to experience the experience of being human. I am here to experience the illusion of separation. I am here to realise the experience is an illusion. I am here to remember I never separated from the source. I am here to experience heaven on Earth.

Wikipedia defines the human body as, "The entire structure of a human being. It is composed of many different types of cells that together create tissues and subsequently organ systems. They ensure homeostasis and the viability of the human body. It comprises a head, neck, trunk (which includes the thorax and abdomen), arms and hands, legs and feet."

Where is the mind? There is no physical location for the mind. In the Oxford English Dictionary the mind is defined as, "The element of a person that enables them to be aware of the world and their experiences, to think, and to feel; the faculty of consciousness and thought."

And the spirit is defined in the Oxford English Dictionary as, "The non-physical part of a person which is the seat of emotions and character."

Science is now showing us that 99.9999% of matter including you and I, is nothing but empty space. How is that possible you ask? Well let me explain. If you remember from your physics class, you learnt about neutrons, protons and electrons which make up what is known as an atom. The neutrons and protons formed together are called a nucleus, which is in the middle, while the electrons fly around in a cloud, kind of like bees.

Now imagine if the nucleus were to be as big as a peanut with the electrons whizzing round. Where would the electrons be? If you thought they would be near your head, you would be wrong. In fact, if the nucleus was as big as a peanut the electrons would be flying around a football stadium. That is how much space there is in between the nucleus and the electrons. And, if you were able to remove all the space in between the nucleus and electrons for all the seven billion people on the planet, we would fit into a single sugar cube. So what does this really mean? The body isn't physical either! We already knew the mind and spirt weren't. But to see in reality, we are nothing physical, so what are we?

Relating these three aspects to the stuttering freedom journey which I call "The Stuttering Triangle."

Mental/Emotional (Mind): 90% Stuttering is an inside job. If you can speak aloud when in your own company, then you know how to speak. So therefore you just have to regulate your breathing and nerves when speaking in front of others. If you cannot speak out aloud when alone without stuttering, then you will first need to work on the physical aspect of the stuttering/blocking so as to convince your mind that you can speak. It's my belief that anyone that doesn't have a physical ailment such as stroke can learn to speak without stuttering. Over time you had learnt to speak in a stuttering way so now you will need to retrain yourself into speaking in a more confident, powerful and eloquent way. It will take discipline, determination and courage. Once you can hear yourself speaking alone then it's time to work on the inner game.

Physical (Body): 10% In any stutterer, the breathing can be noticed as shallow, short, choppy and out of control. When articulating sounds and words, this must be done when breathing correctly.

Spirit: You are not the body. All the great teachers have professed this truth. Jesus said:

"Do you not know that your body is a temple of the Holy Spirit, who is in you, whom you have received from God? You are not your own; you were bought at a price. Therefore honor God with your body," (1 Cor. 6:19-20).

If indeed, like the great teachers have proclaimed we are not the body but indeed spirit, then know this truth "we are all one". We are not separate. How can I be afraid of myself? As a child and adult with a stutter, I couldn't see this truth. Feeling connected to the universe has freed me.

The outer obvious manifestation of stuttering is a direct result of the inner less obvious turmoil.

You will need to:
- work on the beliefs, thoughts, emotions, feelings, perceptions, habits and actions that are holding you back. This will be the focus in Book 2, Awareness of Stuttering Freedom, of The Stuttering Mind series.
- realise that the fears are of the monkey mind constantly chattering.

Our world, according to Dr El March, who I interviewed for my book Rich Thinking, can be divided into three components: mind, body and spirit. Each has its own unique purpose, she says. The spirit is the life force, which is everlasting, unlimited, all-knowing, all-powerful, one with all and invincible. It's also unconditionally loving and fearless.

Our mind creates by the extension of thought, according to March who explains the mind as having a higher and a lower capacity. The higher identifies with spirit; the lower identifies with the body. Mind and spirit are absolutes, they don't know about relative and comparative situations. Further, she says that the human body has no power or cause to create; it takes on any characteristic that the mind assigns it.

The human brain comprises about a hundred billion nerve cells or neurons which are interconnected by trillions of connections. On average, each connection transmits about one signal per second and some of them thousands of signals per second; somehow this is called 'producing thought.'

"Seeing the physical complexity of this, it's really hard to say where it originates and where it ends. It's like asking or trying to find out where the forest begins: is it from the first leaf? Is it from the first root? We really don't know," March says.

"So when we're talking about mind we have the higher and lower minds: internal and external intellect. Our higher and also lower minds are constantly in the give and receive mode. We create thoughts spiritually as well as physically. For us to understand how spiritual thoughts come about, I need to briefly touch on the subject of collective mind. Our higher mind is constantly drying and depositing into the collective mind so some of the thoughts are not even ours but due to the frequency we have created, we receive them."

March offers insight into understanding the lower mind, with a crossed line on a telephone conversation. "The lower minds react to physical stimuli," she says. "And in that, let's say when a feather brushes against your skin or the phone rings; each experience triggers a series of signals in the brain because of their thoughts. But thoughts themselves create a series of reactions due to our belief systems; the same thought in two people creates a completely different reaction."

She continues, explaining, "Our thoughts are also vibrations of energy, we are on autopilot most of the day actually: we work, we converse, we worry, we hope, we plan, we shop, we make love, we play and with all of it we pay minimal attention to how we think. We're basically neglecting this most powerful part of our force in our life."

March says, that this is where using the power of our mind comes in handy, in directing our thoughts towards becoming what is our choice. Our thoughts generate a feeling, and the feelings generate emotions, and the emotions will generate an action or a reaction, so that's how we manifest reality.

Thought for the Day: "The importance of motivation cannot be exaggerated, and success or failure of therapy will depend on your commitment to follow through." Malcom Fraser.

Talking point: Do you really want to make a change in your life and stop stuttering? What will you do to make it happen?

Exercise: Write down in 500 words - In order to live a life free of stuttering you will need to dream it in to existence. What will it take you to reinvent your life? What is stopping you from taking responsibility for your life and the stuttering? Sit down quietly for a few moments and focus on the life you want to live. Write down in as much detail as possible everything you want to happen. From the dream job to the relationships you want. Feel the feelings, hear the sounds, and smell the smells, and visualise the life you want. Do this for every part of your life. Hold this vision in your mind's eye until you truly believe it. Don't allow any negative thoughts or people interfere with the vision for your life. Keep a DO NOT ENTER sign at the door of your mind. Read Rich Thinking - 66 Days to Freedom every day and keep on reading it daily until you can see a change in your life. If you do this and truly believe what you have written and ensuring nothing or no-one else will side track you, your life will be the one you have just written.

DAY 73: STUTTERING PARADOX

Stuttering involves the whole person and not just the speech. In my life the stutter was a manifestation of my personality. Not one to say boo to a goose, I would avoid any attempt to be noticed. The mere attempt in hiding and not accepting the inherent power and greatness of the soul, that part of me that is always connected to the Divine, meant I was suffocating the expression of my true self. Life is a reflection of what is held deeply inside. The world will reflect those beliefs, situations and people around you to help you realise what lessons you need to learn in this lifetime.

It was my deeply held belief that I had nothing important to say. That had built up over a number of years dating back to childhood. The experiences I had a child formed my world. Until I took time to re-evaluate my beliefs and address those beliefs which were disempowering I wasn't going to be able to make a change in my speech and in my life.

It was my belief that once I stopped stuttering I would have a girlfriend. And, I did stop stuttering for 3 months, when I was on a speech therapy program. However, I was still the same person without a girlfriend. I hadn't developed any social skills, I hadn't really learnt the art of flirting and I hadn't transformed as a person, so the stuttering inevitably returned like a bad penny. The stuttering remained my lifelong companion until I went travelling, spoke to as many people as could, asked girls out and dated, read self-development books and finally went after my dream of being an author and speaker.

Low self-esteem, zero confidence and countless limiting beliefs had to be addressed before the outer manifestation of stuttering would dissipate. Most people think they need to cure the stuttering for their lives to suddenly improve, however it's the other way round. Once your life is fulfilling and happy the speech will improve as a by-product. Having a life of purpose gave me the impetus to take action and the stuttering beast went away.

Stuttering is an unconscious pattern of speaking in a manner that isn't easy for the listener or the speaker. It is a pattern that has been developed since the earliest time of speech formation resulting in a manner of speaking that is not conducive to success.

There may be genetic and hereditary factors as well as auditory and motors differences, however with the conscious effort in reprogramming the subconscious mind, speaking without the stuttering behaviour can be established. It takes determination, hard work, positive attitude, self-awareness and above all persistence. In my first book Rich Thinking, I shared the story of Ray Croc, who at the age of 52, founded the McDonalds empire, after buying out the name and brand from the McDonald's brothers. His motto was determination and persistence.

The secret to freeing the subconscious mind from its automatic process of stuttering when speaking, is to take conscious control of the entire speaking process. Speaking involves thought, breathing, vocal cords, articulators, movement of the mouth and jaw, throat, tongue and control of air flow.

Just like learning to drive, a stutterer needs to retrain the subconscious mind to speak in a controlled and purposeful manner. Just like learning to press down on the clutch to switch gears and then the accelerator pedal to drive off, I needed to learn how to breathe and speak at the optimum moment. If not, the car would stumble and stall, bit like stuttering and blocking in a stutterer.

Over years I had built up fears around words and situations. For instance, I could speak and read aloud perfectly well, yet when I was with other people I would be a shrinking violet. From the age of 8, I had learnt that stuttering was bad and something not to be done. The laughter and name calling from other children in school left me traumatised to such an extent I no longer felt free to express myself. I would forever be a worrier. Worried about what children would say or think about me so I would have silent or muted blocks. I was so afraid of stuttering that I couldn't even stutter openly. I was so locked in my stuttering mind that even making a stuttering noise wasn't possible. I was so embarrassed that I would rather be known as the quiet boring one than the s s s s t t tut tut erer. But everyone did know me. When saying my name, I would try R R R R R R a Ra Ra Ra ma. I would force out the word with all the facial contortions that it involved. It wasn't pretty, in fact it was downright ugly. It is said that 1 in 4 stutterers are girls. When teenage girls stutter, the boys think it's cute, especially if the girl is 'hot'; however when a teenage boy stutters other boys laugh. If only, I had met a girl stutterer when I was a teenager. Perhaps then, the perceptions of my stutter may have changed much earlier.

The key to stuttering freedom is to face the stuttering beast head-on. It has been long programmed in the subconscious mind that the stuttering is something bad and is to be avoided at all costs. The only way round this is to reprogram the subconscious mind with a belief that is empowering. Once you have established speaking in a conscious and controlled way then the secret is to stutter in a conscious, controlled and purposeful way. This is to show the subconscious mind that you are no longer regarding stuttering as bad and something to be avoided. It is critical that you embark on this strategy of retraining your mind as soon as you are in control of the speaking process. I would say that controlled, conscious and purposeful stuttering is fundamental in the stuttering freedom journey. How can you truly escape stuttering when you have lived your life fearful of stuttering and not wanted to stutter? It is in the conscious controlled and purposeful stuttering that freedom can be attained.

The brain's primary function is to keep you safe. Its secondary function is the conservation of energy. As a result, to make changes to your subconscious, you are faced with an uphill battle. Once your neuropathways have been created, it takes a great deal of effort and energy to create new ones. However, as a human being, you not only have the ability to experience life, but you are able to be aware or reflect on this experience. You can examine your thoughts, feelings and emotions. You also can imagine how your life could be, under different circumstances. You can dream! Through dreams and goals you can live the life you want. You can do and be anything. You are limitless. The only limitation is not dreaming big enough.

By focusing on what you truly want i.e. living and breathing it, you can bring it into your reality. Your current reality is based on your current beliefs, thoughts and habits. These need to be reset. You also need to upgrade your knowledge and skills. It is through knowledge that you will be empowered; it is through skills that you will achieve; and it is through focus that you will succeed. You are born with the ability to create the life of your dreams.

So, let me ask the same question again: Are you committed or are you just interested? If you are interested you will keep on reading books, going to different speech therapy courses and carry on with your existence. If you are committed you will do whatever it takes to make the changes in your life that you so desire, however radical those changes might be.

If you are committed to the process then the second fundamental strategy in reprogramming the mind is to adopt the process of cancellation. Developed by Charles Van Riper, who was a stutterer himself, it is absolutely vital in your stuttering freedom journey. The subconscious mind stores every single event in your life. In order to reprogram your subconscious mind which, if you remember is there to keep you safe and conserve energy, that will mean your brain will not want to cancel that last situation or word which didn't come out the way you had wanted.

This is a perfectly natural thing. Your mind wants to do the least amount of work. This is where discipline, determination and dedication come in. If you want to become truly free from stuttering then you will need to be disciplined to pull yourself up when you have a stumble in your speech. You need to be your own coach. You will need to build determination into your psyche so it does not become a habit of not cancelling. You will need to be dedicated in your desire to reprogram your mind and become free from the stuttering.

Don't become dependent on any program or someone else. You know when you speech is 'shit'. You know what you need to do to get it back on track. You have been on all the courses that you actually need. You don't need to be a book speech coach with all the knowledge and none of the application. Be your own life speech coach. I know exactly when I am stumbling out of control. I am perfectly aware of what I had just said. I am not drunk and out of my mind. The subconscious mind is the largest database you have. It records everything. Every stumble, every slip up, every time you don't bother to reprogram it with a memory of you saying the word properly. It knows. It is the gatekeeper of your life. Let it slip once, it will remember, Let it slip again, it will remember. Let it slide once more, you will be back in the stuttering jungle before you know it and it will take you 15 years to get out. I speak from experience. I was on a speech therapy programme. I went to repeat 3-day fixes for the high of speaking fluently. I didn't embrace the importance of consciously controlled and purposeful stuttering or the reprogramming of the mind cancellation strategies. I paid the price. 16 wasted years.

Thought for the Day: "Learning how to help yourself should be the goal of every stutterer." Malcolm Fraser.

Talking Point: Why do you think you persisted stuttering when it is said that 4 out of 5 children grow out of stuttering? Are you hypersensitive to the opinion of others, like I was? Do you worry or think a lot about the stuttering throughout the day? Do you think about stuttering before you go to sleep and when you wake up?

Exercise: Go to www.thestutteringmind.com/exercises to download all the exercises that will help you in the quest for freedom.

DAY 74: STUTTERING VOODOO

Stuttering isn't just a speech production problem. It's a problem communicating with others. Most, if not all stutterers can speak and read aloud when alone. It is only in the presence of other people that the stuttering occurs. That was the case with me. I could speak to the cat perfectly well and sang, 'Ding dong bell, pussy in the well,' as I dropped my aunt's cat into the well. She, I mean, the aunt wasn't amused. The cat had 9 lives so lived to tell its tale of how the stuttering boy dropped her in the well.

There seems to be a view held by some that in the dissipation of the stuttering there has to be some voodoo or black magic. My friend, Alex Mandossian, who is known as the Warren Buffet of the Internet, who has made a million dollars in a day, shared the story of the woman and pigeons. When Mandossian, was broke and living at his parent's home he witnessed a life changing event. He was at a park watching how a woman was feeding pigeons. A young boy, maybe aged 6 also saw the pigeons being fed and wanted to do the same. And when the boy held out his hand with bird seed, they didn't approach. What the boy missed, were the steps that the old woman did in getting the first bird to approach. 'You don't ask a girl to marry you on the first date,' Mandossian advised me. I guess that was where I went wrong, when I remained single and dateless for many years. This applies to people who want to make money on the internet. They see people making millions on YouTube and want the same. What they don't see is the hard work behind the scenes. This is exactly the same with stuttering. There is no short cut – no black magic – no voodoo. Facing the fear and doing it anyway is the passport to freedom. It's time to blow away the cobwebs of your limited mind. Do what you are afraid of and you will see it no longer scares you.

Since the time of pioneer, John Harrison, former Associate Director of the National Stuttering Association in the United States, who made his stuttering disappear, he has long advocated the view that stuttering therapy which is primarily focused on controlling the speech isn't the solution. One needs to look at the whole self. His stutter didn't disappear overnight. He evolved from a young boy who stuttered with his friends in the class and yet in the school yard he would speak without any problems, to a man who attended Toastmasters in order to overcome his fear of introducing himself. He literally spent years analysing his whole self and working on blowing away his fears. Everyone wants a short cut. There is no short cut.

After my first intensive 3-day speech therapy course in August 2001, I was on a roller coaster of up and down emotions as the stuttering resurfaced. The stuttering hexagon developed by John Harrison was brought to life, with role plays showing how the whole body is used in the communication process. It was an introduction into the true inner world of stuttering. I was on a high after giving my first public speech in front of 50 people. It was the first time I had spoken in public. My beliefs had just been reset. I have been able to speak in public since that day without any major dramas. One cobweb was blown away. The other one being, "I am no longer afraid of speaking with stutterers so I don't stutter with them." Another cobweb I blew away last year was, "I love stuttering on purpose." I actively do it regularly so it retrains my subconscious mind, telling it – "I am happy stuttering, I am a happy stutter. I am happy stuttering on purpose."

However, it would take another 16 years for the iceberg to melt. There was a point where I learnt while writing my first book, Rich Thinking, that I had to accept full and complete responsibility for everything in my life and to run my own race. This is Law Number 1 of Rich Thinking!

Many years ago, I had read my one and only personal development book, entitled, "Say Yes To Your Potential." Skip Ross, the author, recounted an event where he was attending when a speaker said, "You have right now exactly what you want." That shook Skip then and it shook me as I read it over and over again. As someone whose life wasn't the one I had dreamt of, I had to accept that statement. I was responsible for every thought, feeling and action in my life. It was about taking ownership and personal power and not feeling sorry for myself. I had to re-invent myself as my friend, Allon Khakhouri, former manager of Novak Djokovic, puts it when he talked about Djokovic reinventing himself to become the world number one tennis player after being beaten numerous times by Roger Federer and Rafael Nadal.

Albert Einstein said, "No problem can be solved from the same level of consciousness that created it." For over a century, speech therapists all over the world have attempted to cure stuttering.

Norbert Lieckfeldt, the former CEO of the British Stammering Association said sarcastically in response to a Facebook post, "Yes it's purely psychological. All you have to do is pull yourself together. Now where have I heard this before." As a person who stuttered for over 30 years, there was no indication that the stuttering would dissipate, but indeed it has. At the age of eight I was labelled a stutterer and condemned myself to a life of holding back and avoidance due to negative feedback. As a child I wasn't aware of the inherent greatness within. That has now been rectified. I have started to blow some more of the cobwebs and bring on more challenges.

Albert Einstein quite beautifully said, "A human being is a part of the whole called by us universe, a part limited in time and space. He experiences himself, his thoughts and feeling as something separated from the rest, a kind of optical delusion of his consciousness. This delusion is a kind of prison for us, restricting us to our personal desires and to affection for a few persons nearest to us. Our task must be to free ourselves from this prison by widening our circle of compassion to embrace all living creatures and the whole of nature in its beauty."

Imagine for one millisecond that what Einstein said is true, how we are part of the universe just like the drop of water is part of the ocean. Imagine if the creator gave you its creative power to create your life as your will it, but you forgot it. Einstein is no idiot, so why not believe him?

I quote from my book Rich Thinking... in the Middle Ages witches were burnt at the stake, if I am the stuttering voodoo wizard then so be it. There is an inherent greatness within each and every one of us. Jesus said, "You are all Gods." God created man in his own image and likeness. We have the power to create our reality as we will it.

For those who have been brainwashed by society, it's too late. For those who are reading this and want to know the truth about the matrix, look within your soul. Be silent, be still. The monkey mind that is your companion is just that. It is constantly taking, always criticising, always worrying, never satisfied. It's time to realise you are not your thoughts. Become aware of your thoughts, become conscious of being alive.

It is in the silence that realisation will dawn upon you. You are not your thoughts, you are the observer. You are the very same soul that peered out when you were 8 years old. It's the same soul that looked out when you were 18. It's the same soul that is reading this at this very moment. You are not the body that had gone through a lifetime of experiences; you are the everlasting spirt that is connected to everyone and everything. You are Divine.

You have a choice right now. Accept responsibility for the life you lead. No else had made you hold back and avoid speaking situations. It's not about blame, it's about personal power. You can choose to have the power and work on your inner game to get the freedom you so desire.

If you can speak without stuttering in one situation then you can speak in any situation. This maybe a hard pill to take but the truth of it is you have chosen to speak like this. It is your subconscious mind that is making the choice. Consciously you want to speak but years of negative feedback and programming has led your subconscious resisting your conscious efforts that results in the stuttering and blocking. If stuttering has a physical basis, then why is former US Vice President Joe Biden not stuttering. Once a stutter, always a stutter is not the case. Look at Ed Sheeran, Bruce Willis and the countless others who have made the stutter disappear. It is in the belief of what is possible and impossible your reality is created. If Ed Sheeran had stood still and didn't rap to Eminem lyrics then he would be known as Stuttering Ed instead of the amazingly genius singer song writer he is.

The mind is the most powerful gift given by the creator. With your mind you can choose to relive the horror stories of stuttering or have visions of speaking in front of thousands. Whatever you put into your mind you will create.

If you are happy with the stutter then stop reading stuttering blogs and remove yourself from stuttering Facebook groups. If you want to stop stuttering then take charge, accept your personal power that you have the ability to transform. Resolve to do whatever it takes. Start reading personal development books and spend time with people who have made the stutter disappear. Above all, believe in yourself and find the inner knowing that you are the Divine experiencing itself on this Earthly plane. Remember to ask yourself, why is it that I can speaking perfectly well when I am alone and yet when I am in front of others I block and stutter. What part of me, isn't comfortable expressing itself to others.

Thought for the Day: "I thought I was handicapped. I couldn't talk at all. I still stutter around some people now." Bruce Willis

Talking point: Bruce Willis says he still stutters around some people. Do you think he let his stuttering behaviour rule his life? He has been one of the most successful actors in recent times. It doesn't really matter if you stutter. If you think of it as a plight on your life then it will be. If you live your life irrespective of the stutter then you will see that the stuttering will disappear.

Exercise: Go to www.thestutteringmind.com/exercises to download all the exercises that will help you in the quest for freedom.

DAY 75: THE TRUTH

lbert Einstein is quoted as saying, "Insanity is doing the same thing, over and over again, but expecting different results." I think I must have gone insane. I had attended an intensive 3-day speech therapy course, and over the subsequent years I attended even more courses in the attempt to break free from stuttering. I was living my own groundhog day. I would struggle with the speech, go back on courses and struggle again. The constant battle with the failure of progressing despite the hours of physical and mental effort resulted in depression and the final realisation that it wasn't going to work out for me. If I need to make a breakthrough, it would have to be on my own.

In my book *Rich Thinking - 66 Days to Freedom*, my friend Chris Payne shares what Mark Anastasi, New York Times best-selling author of the Laptop Millionaire told him, "Many years ago, Mark said to me that success online is 90% mindset. I agree. He said, 'Here's the thing, Chris: if I run a course on the latest online success techniques, I can fill a room with hundreds of people who want to take part. But if I run a mindset course because mindset is 90% of making money, I only get a couple of dozen people.' I thought it was very profound of Mark to say that."

This insight helped shape my journey to stuttering freedom. If indeed making money online is 90% mindset, then without a doubt stuttering is also 90% mindset. As a person who stuttered, I was constantly thinking about my speech, and whether or not it would hold up in the world outside the stuttering community. I wanted to speak beyond techniques and enjoy connecting with people without the voice in the head. In the course of setting out to interview 20 people to write my first book, it proved quite difficult. Once I changed my mind-set and really believed it was possible for me to get interesting people and interview them, I got the rest very easily. I had read about Ollie Forsyth, a young man who was dyslectic and he had been bullied at school. Now, aged 19, he runs The Budding Entrepreneur Club helping people network. He was the first person I interviewed. Initially I was nervous and told people about the stutter beforehand, but in subsequent interviews, I just spoke and was myself. After reviewing the interviews, I realised that I did not stumble over words that much and was feeling elated at how they went. I was on my way to freedom after pursing my dream.

If stuttering is 90% in the mind then the struggles I had been having was due to my thinking. Whenever I had a stumble in my speech, I would build it up to mean such a big life changing event, so that resulted in a life time of stuttering. I would follow the rules of the speech therapy program by going out, talking to strangers and working on the challenging words. This was all well and good, however when it really counted the speech was shocking.

Quite a number of people who stutter aren't honest with themselves or with others who are on the same journey. I count myself as one of these people. I would attend courses and support meetings, project myself as someone whose speech was at a good level, where in fact the speech was all but. This falsehood would persist over a number of years. It was a case of not wanting to lose face with the others in the group. I now believe the majority of people who are struggling with their speech, who are part of a group have to deal with this elephant in the room. The case of wanting to be fluent in the real world had been transferred to the stuttering world. For me, speaking without stuttering at stuttering community events meant a release from the years of sitting on the sidelines. I was now in a situation where I would be stutter free. I was no longer giving my power to anyone, but it was only in this scenario. With the non-stuttering world, I was a like a rabbit in front of a fox. Stuttering for me is a habit that I held on to for so many years. It isn't an easy journey, simply attending a 3-day intensive course. There is no quick fix. Since it took me many years to learn that stuttering is bad, it has taken me a long time to unlearn it.

It was meeting Simon, on one such course, that illuminated my path. He and I quickly became friends. He too, was an IT contractor, so sharing an interest in technology and speech, meant we had lots to talk about. He was about 18 years older. He reminded me of another friend, Roger, who I had first met on another speech therapy course years earlier. But Simon was different. He had been married and had 3 kids. He was living his life despite the stutter. Simon and I would discuss why our speech would fluctuate so much. I knew I could speak beyond techniques to other stutterers. I was completely relaxed. I really enjoyed talking and conversing with people who stutter, but when it came to talking to non-stutters I would experience a brain freeze and not have anything much to say. I was stuck in the mindset of a stutterer and constantly worried about my speech so wasn't able to let go and be free to express myself. Simon soon left the world of IT and went into to setting up a hypnotherapy practise. I was impressed at how far he had progressed with his speech. He is Mr No Holding Back.

The reality of the journey is it is a long term game. A 3-day intensive course teaching breathing techniques and mostly the physical aspects of speaking does not cut it. In reality stuttering is an inside job and I needed to take responsibility for my life and speech. The outer obvious manifestation of stuttering is a direct result of a less obvious inner turmoil. I had to re-invent myself just like Novak Djokovic.

Law number one in Rich Thinking is to accept responsibility for everything in your life and run your own race. Stop blaming others. Stop making excuses. You created your world with your thoughts, emotions, feelings, perceptions, habits, beliefs and actions. You have the power to change now. Don't compare yourself to others; just strive to be the best you can.

Apart from a few close friends who were on the journey to stuttering freedom, I dropped out of the speech therapy world. I didn't see a need to attend courses or support meetings again, especially when I knew the speech would be perfect in those situations.

After many years of not meeting stutterers I met Ramesh. He lived close to me and we met for the first time in Stevenage, when he came to help me at my book stall. I then realised there were people who stuttered who were on a similar journey. They had become disillusioned with traditional speech therapy methods and found freedom.

I then met Ruban, the second ever Sri-Lankan Tamil person who stuttered. 30 years previously I met Jehan, who stuttered. He was a young man who lived in Manchester and when he met me, he started laughing. Jehan told me he started stuttering because he was imitating one of his classmates. Ruban is the man behind the awesome motivational videos at Stutterhacks.

I met Alex, a Russian businessman who had lived in the United States, before moving to London. He too had a stutter and attended a 3-day intensive course. However he was getting out there, making a name for himself as FindingVoices99 and doing podcasts along with Eugene and Tom. They hadn't let the stutter rule their lives.

I also met a Nigerian businessman, Ayo, who was suicidal before he found his voice. Having attended a personal development seminar he also realised that stuttering is an inside job. He is the man behind Stop Holding Back along with Chris.

They all are my stuttering posse.

People want tactics and strategies. They want sexy, quick and easy techniques to make money. They want to make money doing nothing. And there are people who will sell you this idea. The concepts vary from stock trading to real estate and from currency trading to selling on EBay. There are many who go after the shiny new objects, however they will never taste success. They go from one course to another and end up wasting their time and money. This also relates to stuttering.

Everyone wants to speak without stuttering. They want to be just like the other non-stutters. I include myself in this. I wanted to be 'cured' within 3 days of intensive speech therapy. I wanted that magic red pill. However there is no pill. It's an inner journey of discovery that was the key to freedom. In Rich Thinking you can create a habit of reading. It has 66 chapters that are divided into days. Reading one chapter will take you between 5 and 10 minutes. With a thought for the day, talking points and exercises you can download and complete you will be on the road to freedom.

Essentially, speaking is a simple process but has been made complicated by the stuttering mind. Most of the world does it subconsciously without any effort, just like walking. Imagine you have a baby and he fell over. When he fell over, you picked him up quickly, so as to reassure him you will be there. He falls over again, and you just fail to catch him this time and he starts crying. The next time he tries a few steps, he falls again and cries. Seeing that it was the third time, he fell over, the baby will become cautious and hold on to a rail or table to give himself support. He would quickly move along the room as long as there was a wall or table for support. And when walking outside he would hold your hand. By now, it has been engrained in his subconscious mind, that if he lets go of your hand he will fall over. So he has a hard time letting go. Now imagine this same baby is 6 years old and falling over and needing a hand to go anywhere and not able to walk without a hand of support. I have never seen this happen. I can't imagine a 6 year old going to school needing to be hand held all the time so as not to fall over. The parents quite rightly encouraged the baby to make baby steps and start walking. However in the case of a child who has a stutter, for whatever reason, the subconscious didn't learn how to co-ordinate the activities needed in order to produce speech effectively. And in this case, the parents, didn't know how to help their child to speak without fear or apprehension. Parents can only do their best. It is a common occurrence for toddlers to stumble over words as they begin to learn to communicate. For some, speech therapy helps but for us adult stutterers, we kept hold of this way of speech production. Stuttering is a complex psychological issue that has layers upon layers like an onion. At some point I had developed self-doubt in my ability to produce sounds and words. This lead to a fear of stuttering when speaking. After a while this resulted in avoiding words. Later on it would be an avoidance of situations. And many years later it would mean sitting on the sidelines and avoiding life. Depression and suicidal thoughts would cross my mind.

Thought for the Day: "The happiest stutterers, I learned, are those who are willing to stutter in front of others." John Stossel

Talking point: Do you go from one speech therapy course to another speech therapy course searching for the next fix of fluency. It's time to take responsibility and start to practice conscious controlled and purposeful stuttering. The mind cannot differentiate between what is imagined and real, so practice in your mind's eye or practice in front of the mirror. Then practice in front of people who you are totally comfortable around. You will then see and feel that there is no shame attached to stuttering. The negative emotions will slowly dissipate over time as you being to take control over the stuttering pattern that had previously ruled your life.

Exercise: Go to www.thestutteringmind.com/exercises to download all the exercises that will help you in the quest for freedom.

If you want those sexy quick techniques to help you immediately then email me with the subject: Sexy Speech Techniques at hellorama@thestutteringmind.com and I will add you to an exclusive group.

DAY 76: THE BRAIN REPAIRS STUTTERING

S tutterers see stuttering as bad and something to be stopped at all costs. In the process of wanting to stop the behaviour, this desire to stop causes a resistance. This resistance results in the continued manifestation of the behaviour, in this case the stutter persists despite the conscious mind's resolve in stopping the stutter. It is only when the subconscious mind is in alignment with the goals of the conscious that freedom beckons. To define stuttering as evil or bad, still holds an emotional charge. The stutter served its purpose, the behaviour may have protected you as a child, for which you need to be thankful for. It's only in the gratitude of having a stutter can one release the demons of the life experienced as a result of the stutter. It is easy to say this with the benefit of hindsight of stuttering freedom, but this is the path. To continue to hold the thought that stuttering is bad will result in the continued manifestation of the stutter.

The outer world is a reflection of the inner world. It is in the inner world that your reality is created. Beliefs that have been moulded over time have made the life you have. Just look around you to see what beliefs you hold. Where you live and the life you lead are manifested according to your beliefs. These beliefs lie in your subconscious mind. You are not consciously aware of them, which is why however much you try to do something, it just seems out of reach.

A stutterer who has lived a long life of stuttering has probably never examined the possibility of the above being possible. Just suppose, a trauma caused the stutter, and in that moment the child with its limited knowledge, processed it to mean that its life was being threatened. In the past, when a sabre-toothed tiger was strolling by in the jungle, the threat was obvious. But now where stress is known as the black plague of the 21st century, threats are not as obvious. Cortisol streams through your body whenever you are stressed, and as a stutterer you are stressed most of the time.

Recent research suggests that stuttering is caused by activity in the brain being different to non-stutterers. To produce speech, the combined correct coordination of breathing, movement of the throat, tongue and lips are necessary for sounds and words to be produced. This involves various parts of the brain and it appears in MRI scans that people who stutter have missing neuro connections.

However, I am of the belief it is the stuttering that has caused these missing connections. This is the chicken or egg question. Which came first? If this was the case then former US Vice President Joe Biden should still be stuttering. And everyone who had a stutter will continue their life of stuttering. If you, had the chance of reading Rich Thinking, you will have developed the habit of reading for 66 days. New neuropathways would have been formed in your brain. Neuroplasticity is the superpower we are born with. By adopting practices to control your mind and thoughts you can do the impossible.

Dr. Christian Kell, is a neuroscientist from the Brain Imaging Centre, Frankfurt in Germany, who published a research paper in 2009 entitled 'How the brain repairs stuttering'. Starting in 2005, the team scanned the brains of 13 adult male stutterers, who stuttered from their childhood using functional magnetic resonance imaging, while reading out aloud German sentences, before and after fluency shaping therapies. They also scanned 13 males who had recovered from stuttering without any form of therapy and another 13 males who were the control subjects.

Dr Kell explained, "The idea was to look at the functional correlates of what this therapy actually changes in the brain and we compared this activity to the brain activities of fluent people who stutter and also to 13 male participants who used to stutter for years but have stopped stuttering without any, well let's say causal-therapy, spontaneous recovery."

It was observed, "if we compared people who stutter, their brain activity during speaking, with the brain activity of fluent speakers, we observed something that is often seen in many imaging studies on stuttering that you actually see an over activation of the right hemisphere."

Elaborating further, "So, usually the left half of the brain, is the part of the brain that is able to produce speech fluently. We basically confirmed this over recruitment of the right hemisphere, the right half in the brain in those participants."

However, he did note, "those who were moderate to severely stuttering speakers, in the scanner in the social isolation in the board and maybe also due to auditory masking, because you have this constant scanner noise around, all the participants were fluent so, even if you have a severe stutter, inside the scanner usually participants do not stutter and this is maybe surprising."

This reminded me of when Mushy from the British TV program, Educating Yorkshire, listened to music on headphones while speaking in front of his classmates and he didn't stutter at all. Could this provide a clue in giving relief to other stutterers?

Adding Dr Kell said, "this is actually something that we wished for. That's a good condition for us, as researchers because we can compare the brain activity during quasi-similar overt behavior. We know that it is not completely identical, but still I think it's a comparable behavior and that any change in brain activity is rather related to the path of physiology or the compensation for stuttering. And so, I think the advantages is that we are not looking at different states and examine how the brain looks during a stutter, but rather how does it look without an overt stuttering behavior in comparison to someone who is not at all stuttering usually."

Explaining how the investigation was conducted focusing on fluency shaping therapy he says, "the speech tempo is rather reduced during therapy, where the speech prosody is drastically altered and I think one of the targets of the therapy is really to change the way of speaking on the behavior level."

Adding, Dr Kell says, "This Kassel stutter therapy is quite successful and I think it was a 2 weeks intensive course, followed by regular refresher courses with even online courses and refresher training."

Elaborating of this further, he said, "this fluency shaping therapy is quite successful in most of the participants to really reduce the stuttering frequencies of the percent of stuttered syllables to below to 2%, which is really excellent, and so what we observed is that this right hemispheric over activation that we see in people who had not yet received such a therapy. So, quazi therapy naïve participants that this over activation was drastically reduced and due to the therapy program and lateralized back to the left hemisphere which is the physiology half of the brain that usually produces speech and so I think this we reported in 2009 in the spring paper. "

He added that when he recently re-analyzed the data and looked at the functional connectivity, the interaction between the brain regions he observed, "that this re-lateralization of the activity to the left hemisphere was associated with a change in functional connectivity between the regions that process the auditory feedback of what just has been produced and the motor control, let's say motor regions in the brain so what we observed was, that people who stutter have reduced interaction between the feedback processing regions and the motor regions that actually are relevant in producing speech and this fits nicely, I think, with lots of other studies who have shown that people who stutter may have deficits in auditory motor interactions."

He continues saying, "So not even only verbal, but maybe, also nonverbal auditory motor interactions that could be disturbed in people who stutter. So there is one inferential idea that auditory feedback is important in stuttering, and this was a nice or an interesting observation to see, that indeed and people who stutter have their reduced functional connectivity between the auditory and the motor context and what we observed now linked to this therapy program was that the connectivity between auditory region and motor regions was improved after therapy, but notable not between those regions that were functionally altered in the people who stuttered before therapy but rather in neighboring regions, so this was particularly the regions that usually associated with feedback processing of slower auditory features."

Explaining, he says, "So it seems that people who stutter may have a reduced auditory motor mapping between regions that are important in processing fast changes in the auditory signal and our data suggested that this therapy program that actually slows down speech is able to recruit a connection between regions that are more involved in controlling those slower speech features and please note that during the scanning itself the participants spoke quasi-equally and if you look at the controls and even the people who stutter, so there was no real behavior overt difference. So that's interesting. So training obviously with reduced speech tempo may help the brain to repair itself."

Neuroplasticity is the superpower that we all have but "it doesn't come out of the blue," says Dr Kell. Continuing he says, "Neuroplasticity is something that you can actually train. So, I think this intensive course helped participants to actually tap into a plasticity mechanism that seems to be available to most of the people who stutter."

He explains, "If you look at the average response you actually see this re-lateralization to the left half of the brain activity during speech production, associated with the recruitment of those regions, who have actually much slower speech features even if you don't speak slowly anymore. So it seems that training with reduced speech tempo may help people who stutter to actually recruit those plasticity mechanism."

When I explained to Dr Kell about my journey to stuttering freedom, I learnt when I was with other people who stuttered I was 'fluent' more, I was okay, I was myself. I didn't stutter because in my own mind I was comfortable, I was not being judge by them and I was free to be myself, to express myself. So, I had no real tension but in the next second if I was with a fluent speaker, my speech would fall apart.

Dr Kell commented, "I think there is for sure there is an important psychological component to stuttering and I did my post-doctoral work in Paris and you may know that in France, psychoanalyst are actually pretty important and they have a huge psycho analytical culture there and we have a very interesting debate on the question of those psychological symptoms secondary to neurobiological problem or that was their view - is everything we see in brain scans for example - is that simply a consequence of psychological trauma before?"

Continuing he adds, "And so obviously it's very difficult to disentangle that and I think we have a pretty good evidence now also from genetics that there is a genetic component to stuttering. We have pretty good evidence, I think that may be a primary neurobiological problem that leads to stuttering but the interesting argument is, so if you speak for example to a psychoanalyst, how can you be sure that whatever you observed even in stuttering kids is not already a consequence of a psycho trauma. So, we cannot entirely be sure that a psychological trauma can also contribute for example to stuttering and I would not at all rule that out." Which came first, the chicken or the egg?

Going on further he says, "On the other hand I would argue against this notion that stuttering is a psychological or purely psychiatric disorder, I would definitely disagree on that. I think it is a pretty good evidence for a neurobiological reason for stuttering. You are not at all alone with the notion if you are, for example in more demanding situations, emotional situations that your stutter would become more intense and a very straight forward interpretation would be that your brain already always tries to compensate. Imagine you have a neurobiological deficit, so let's simplify now and say you have a deficit in auditory motor mapping and so the brain tries to compensate for that and so we know that the right brain tries to assist and tries to help out to reduce stuttering but the problem is it does not seem to lead to a full recovery. "

Explaining, Dr Kell says, "Because otherwise people would not continue stuttering. So the regions that we see there, that are activated in people who stutter that have not yet had a therapy, those regions belong to so called control network. This control network in the brain is important to everything you're doing. You need this control network if you plan your holidays and you think about what you still have to work on. In these things you need this network and if you use this network in part also to compensate for stuttering, it seems clear that your resources may be limited and in case you are engaged in more difficult tasks for example, then your stuttering would become more severe because your compensation mechanism are used for something else and there's for sure also a huge emotion component. So if you become emotional about your speech then this may not be helpful at all because you attribute fear and negative values to something that is usually automatized."

Dr Kell does not believe that stuttering could be a learned behavior, for example a habituated way of speaking with sound and word repetitions, built up over a period of years the adult stutterer continues that way of speaking subconsciously. However, he says, "I'm pretty sure that stuttering events by themselves, elicit learning, I absolutely agree. If you experience more and more stuttering events, this will have negative connotation for example and you may learn this association between speaking and negative emotions and this in turn may have consequences for your way of speaking. So yes there will be learning components but I don't believe that stuttering by itself is something that someone has learned."

Relating this to the people who have who recovered spontaneously in adulthood. Dr Kell explains, "You may know that most of the kids who actually have disfluencies during the speech development, not just physiological ones but actually stuttering and they recover early on also during their childhood but now a couple of people who stutter into adulthood lose their stutter in a couple of months or years."

He goes on to share, "what we observed is the role of the cerebellum, which is the part of the brain that is primary involved in controlling coordination and what we observed was that people that recovered from stuttering during adulthood they actually disconnect part of the superior cerebellum from the speech production network and interestingly through a region that is evolved also in the effective evaluation of behavior. So we found this orbital frontal cortex being important to recovering and so it seems that this orbital frontal cortex is differently involved in speech production in people who recovered from stuttering compared from people who stutter and this was actually the only region that significantly disassociated people who still stutter from people who recovered from their stuttering and the role that we believe this change place is a different emotional evaluation of the act of speaking and interestingly it may have to do, we are not yet sure about this, it may have to do with the evaluation of the auditory compared to the somatosensory feedback. So it seems that until you did not fix the auditory motor mapping, you rely more on the somatosensory feedback of the feeling of your mouth for producing speech and after therapy and after such a spontaneous recovery for example it seems that the auditory feedback or the importance of the auditory feedback is restart."

Relating whether stuttering runs in families, he says," you see that there is a stronger relationship with stuttering in identical twins compared to non-identical twins and this clearly shows you that there is a genetic component."

As to why a lot of children, when they are 3 or 4 spontaneously recover, and then the tiny minority hold on to this stuttering that develops Dr Kell says, "that is a very important question, we don't have the answer yet and it may be that they have a different genetic background, it may be that they have different neuroplasticity mechanisms available. It may be that they have a different way of coping with it and so for example they have different learning and compared to the other kids who recover. But I, at least to my knowledge, I'm not aware of individual factors that have been identified that will make the distinction. I'm pretty sure that there is really old work already on the analysis of speech signals itself, I think even there you cannot associate clearly which kid is going to recover and which other kid is going to continue stuttering so if you ask me, I'm pretty sure it will be a mixture of all those effects so maybe some other genetic backgrounds, maybe some other neuroplastic mechanisms and maybe also other ways to cope and deal with stuttering symptoms."

Much of the speaking process is subconscious, or "automatized" as Dr Kell puts it. "The act of speaking is clearly conscious," however, "the muscle reflexes and the exact articulation most of that is not conscious." Dr Kell explains further saying, "the standard way of speaking is a conscious one. Including all the automatized processes that are below and most of them are unconscious, I absolutely agree but I would, so far for example breathing is very different. Breathing is really an automatized motor behavior and obviously continues during sleep. I would argue that you would not usually speak during sleeping, but I agree that there are exceptions."

Concluding, Dr Kell says, "I'm pretty sure that those emotional aspects have an impact on speaking because if you start getting afraid of the act of speaking itself, you will run into difficulties. So this over emphasis and maybe the wish to perfectly be fluent, this may not always be for everybody a good recipe."

Thought for the Day: "The stream of knowledge is heading towards a non-mechanical reality; the universe begins to look more like a great thought than a great machine. Mind no longer appears to be an accidental intruder into the realm of matter, we ought rather to hail it as the creator and governor of the realm of matter. Get over it and accept the inarguable conclusion. The universe is immaterial–mental and spiritual." Sir James Jeans

Talking point: Do you talk when you are asleep? And if so, do you stutter? Do you remember your dreams? Are you stuttering in your dreams?

DAY 77: THREE MONTHS

I clearly remember the decision of enrolling on yet another speech therapy course. It had been a few years since the goldfish and gerbil tape that I religiously practiced speaking out loud to whilst I was driving. It was 2 months after I had started working at the Prime Minister's Office. My speech was atrocious. I felt ashamed and embarrassed. I was 25 years old and I was an out of control train wreck of a stutterer.

All semblance of the speech technique that I used when I was in college 7 years previously had disappeared. I was truly and utterly lost in the stuttering jungle. My mother had heard about the speech therapy course when I was 21 but at nearly a $1000 it was too much money to spend on yet another course that may or may not have worked.

I had stuttered since the age of 8, and like any other child I had stumbled over words when speaking since I was a toddler, but that was the age I was labelled as a stutterer and was sent to speech therapy. I was in class and was reading aloud. I can't say for certain how I was feeling at that moment in time, but I am confident that stuttering wasn't a word in my vocabulary. I was just an eight-year-old boy reading aloud in class.

I was learning to read aloud and yet the label of stutterer had just been imprinted on my mind. This label has been stuck on my psyche for over 30 years and 2017 is the year I broke free. So what if I stutter, I am in great company, Moses, Aristotle, Charles Darwin, Lewis Carroll, to name just a few. Looking back at history the impact these people who had a speaking challenge didn't stop them from leading their lives, so now it's my turn.

I read with interest that Lewis Carroll suffered from a bad stutter, but he found himself vocally fluent when speaking with children. So obviously there was nothing wrong in his speaking process. He could quite clearly speak in front of young children and so it was he wrote Alice's Adventures in Wonderland, after an afternoon picnic with Alice and her 2 sisters. If Lewis Carroll could speak in one situation, he could have spoken well in all situations, if only he had read Rich Thinking!

For 25 years the pain of stuttering wasn't big enough. Yes I was ashamed and embarrassed by the way I spoke, and yet I struggled through. I had periods of depression and felt isolated over that time. Suicidal thoughts even crossed my mind. But I hadn't died. I may have wished to but the thought of doing the deed didn't overrule the pain of stuttering. I think the pain of suicide was greater than the comfort of stuttering.

When I was 18 I had attended a two week intensive speech therapy course at the Lister Hospital in Stevenage. That helped me get some control over my speech but being really honest with myself the pain wasn't that big enough as the stuttering habit persisted until I was 25. I was a comfortable stutterer. I was ok. I was still alive.

There was nothing that made me sit up and make a decision to do something about it, until I was 25 years old and couldn't say a single word to my boss. Philip was dyslectic but that didn't stop him from becoming the Head of IT at the Prime Minister's Office. He once told us that he barged in and saw the Prime Minister in his underwear when he was working on the computers in the home of the First family.

Philip was an interesting character. He was a security guard that studied archaeology. He got a job at No10, only to later find his boss Robin was migrating to New Zealand. So he then found himself being the man in charge of the red button. What made me stutter uncontrollably with Philip was beyond belief. Philip didn't make eye contact with people. He would continue typing away while I spoke to him and the lack of attention caused me to feel rushed and stutter.

The stutter was out of control, it had taken over my life. I was blocking and repeating sounds and words like a parrot. I stuttered and blocked on the phone. I would make sounds from a Freddy Kruger nightmare just to get the words out. And part of my job would be to answer the telephone and help staff with their computer problems so speaking was a necessity.

Now, the stuttering was contextual, in some situations I would manage to speak but it wasn't pretty, in fact it looked pretty ugly with all of my facial contortions, tics and panic expressions at the worst of times. I was a rabbit in headlights, only in my case I was being run over every day.

In August 2001, I enrolled on an intensive 3-day speech therapy program. Sitting waiting on the first day wasn't filled with nerves. I was 25 years old and in a room full of stutterers from all walks of life. The stutter didn't discriminate. Looking at all these people, you wouldn't think they had a deep dark secret, and yet when they opened their mouths, their secret would be instantly exposed. I felt at ease.

The last time I was in a group setting similar to this was when I was 18 years old. That feels like a lifetime ago. I was a complete stutterer. I was with 4 other men at my local hospital. I had just finished my end of school exams and was not looking forward to the results. The stutter had won and I had given up on life. The course was for 2 weeks, and meant staying overnight and returning home at the weekend. I was completely immersed in the speech therapy. At the age of 18, I wasn't comfortable at all, even with stutterers. I was the youngest of the group and felt uneasy and nervous. The intervening seven years resulted in a bit more confidence and composure, however the stutter was still prevalent in my life.

Then I was called up. I honestly couldn't remember how it went. It certainly wasn't as bad as some of the others. There was one guy called Lucatoni who struggled so badly his whole body shook as he spoke. It was unbelievable. There we tongue trusts, fist clenches, head jerks, the works. He was the worst stutterer I have ever seen. It made Ken Pile, the star from the hit 1988 movie of A fish called Wanda, look fluent.

At the end of the first long day, all the new students of the program had to get up and say their name. My heart was pounding as I watched on. One by one the students said their name and it was finally my turn. I got up and breathed. I said 'R' and let the air go out of my lungs. I went for it again, 'Ra' and let the air expel from my lungs again. I tried once again, 'Rama Siva.' I said my name for the first time in front of a group of people without stuttering. I had never done that before. Since the age of eight I had struggled to say my name. Just saying your own name is one of the biggest challenges for many stutterers. And I succeeded. Next up was Lucatoni. He stood up and after a couple of tries he said his name without any drama. It was a total and complete transformation. He said his name without any of the physical and body movements that he previously displayed.

After three days, where I re-learnt how to breath, produce sounds and words, I was in my element. My speech pattern had been reprogrammed. New software had been installed into my conscious mind. Just like learning to drive I had re-learnt how to speak.

I got up on a soap box in Bournemouth and said my name in front of 50 people in the town centre. I had just realised, when I was the centre of attention and knew people were waiting for me to speak I could deliver. I was proud of how far I came. I would like to say that I didn't look back, but life isn't like that.

It was only 16 years later when I went on BBC radio that true liberation was felt. Over the years I wondered if I was ever going to stop stuttering. I went on repeat speech therapy courses like an addict searching for his next fix.

That insight of being able to speak in public would prove to be key in my quest for freedom. In all my speaking situations where I found myself stuttering it would be where I had the feeling of being rushed or felt as if not being paid attention to. I would later be able to do presentations and public speeches without any major worries. When I knew people were listening I could speak without stuttering. However, when I was in a one on one situation or in small groups, I would stutter uncontrollably and be the proverbial wall flower. I hadn't yet worked on my inner game to become truly free.

I was lucky that the Prime Minister's Office paid for the speech therapy course. It was too expensive for me at that time. Many would think the same but what price could you put for freedom. If there was a course that taught me what I have learnt over the last two years and given me lifelong freedom I would gladly pay $10,000. I know, I can earn that amount in a month.

Real freedom has taken 16 years and now I am free. After interviewing 20 entrepreneurs to write my first book entitled Rich Thinking I am free from the holding back, free from negative self-talk, free from the small thinking of what's really possible. I am a drop of water in the ocean that is experiencing itself as the drop. I am the creator of my reality and am thankful for being able to choose the experiences.

Going on BBC radio for the first time wiped 30 years of hurt, sharing with the world my pain was liberating, and hopefully inspiring millions to realise the inner God within them - my mission in life is clear.

Taking action is the key to being free. By making the decision to do something about the stutter, I took the first step. The stutter was a habit that I developed and kept hold off. It was my comfort zone, I was used to speaking in this manner and so it stayed with me. It wasn't until the pain of stuttering was so big that I did something about it.

I had muddled through life. I was getting by but wasn't pursuing my dream of being an author and speaker. It was only when I started interviewing and writing that I assimilated all the insights that I had come across. Realising these universal truths helped me become the person I was meant to be.

I remember, two days after returning home from the speech therapy course crying on my own at the wasted years. I had spent my entire 25 years avoiding life. I had avoided asking girls out for fear of rejection. I had let the stutter take over my life. I had died.

And truth be told, after this course, I was still avoiding life. I was Mr Avoid. Yes I had control over the stutter but the stutter was controlling my life. I would stutter uncontrollably and then go on yet another course. I was like a recovering alcoholic going to AA meetings.

Three months after my first course, I had a stuttering ambush. I was in trouble. I had been doing the breathing exercises, ritually every day, making phone calls and talking with people. However I had a big problem. I went along to my second speech therapy course and got my confidence back up and was flying once again. This time, about three weeks later, I was back in trouble. I made use of the support therapy phone list, but that was now my comfort zone. I soon realised that I never stuttered with people who have a stutter. That was an interesting insight in my journey. For the first time in my life, I could speak to a group of people who have a similar speaking habit as me, without any fear at all. So I went on my third course, fourth course and then I lost count. I was addicted to attending speech therapy courses and the high I would get after speaking with discipline for three days. Every time I got home I would feel absolutely physically and mentally exhausted.

Ten years on after my first course on the speech therapy programme, the pain of stuttering had again finally taken its toll, and after years of still avoiding life, even though the stutter was under control, I was stuck in a rut. I was successful in my business career but my personal and social life was non-existent. I was dying again. I made a decision and went to Madrid to study Spanish. I was motivated for the first time to go towards pleasure.

It had been a dream of mine to travel to South America, but I had been too scared to travel on my own in a continent far away from home. The last time I had travelled to a different continent, was to Australia and the speech was terrible. I avoided situations, people and didn't enjoy the experience. I felt alone. This time I had a purpose. I had booked a two month Spanish language course so I knew I would have my time full and would be forced to speak.

I was out of my comfort zone. But it didn't matter; I enjoyed meeting new people and making new friends. I was still the shy timid boy of 15 as I hadn't developed socially but I was actually having fun. I really enjoyed the experience of being in a classroom. It wasn't the same painful experience I had as a teenager; I was with adults who were all on a journey learning Spanish.

Children can be oh so cruel, if only they knew what they do and say to others would make a lifelong impression then they would be kinder. Richard Branson talks about how his mother taught him to treat others like how he wanted to be treated, and if he didn't, his mother would make him stand in front of the mirror and look at himself. I wish all mothers would do the same, then the world would be full of billionaires and as kind as Branson.

The pleasure of stuttering freedom had enveloped me. After going on BBC radio for the first time I was motivated to continuously blow the cobwebs of my stuttering mind. I was on a mission and that was to show my subconscious that there was nothing more to be feared. The insights I assimilated in writing my book seeped into my subconscious. I was no longer the same person. I was free to express myself as a person who had a stutter and may very well stumble over a few words here and there but did not need to be labelled as a stutterer.

The motivation of being an author and speaker spurred me on to email and chase down people I wanted to interview. It had been a dream of mine to become a bestselling author and as a by-product the stutter dissipated.

What is your motivation in wanting not to stutter? It can be going towards an experience that is pleasurable or one that avoids pain. If you can decide that the experience of stuttering no longer serves you and you are pursuing your dreams then the stutter will be a non-issue. However if you are looking to simply avoid the pain of stuttering then it may very well remain your life companion.

Thought of the Day: "I am you, you are ME, You are the waves; I am the ocean. Know this and be free, be divine." Satya Sai Baba

Talking point: What is your motivation for not stuttering? Are you actually comfortable living the life of a stutterer?

DAY 78: AMBUSHED

It was about three months after my first speech therapy course, I was ecstatic and my speech and confidence levels were sky high. I had taken the opportunity to disclose to Alastair Campbell, the former press secretary to Prime Minister Tony Blair, that I was working to overcome my stuttering. He was amazing about it and told me 'Well done.' Years later, I read that he suffered from depression from time to time. Wow, even the greatest spin doctor is human!

And then it occurred. It was just a random event, I was explaining to a colleague something related to my job and I had a block on a word. In that moment I experienced my first stuttering ambush, and all the hard work I had done went up in smoke. I struggled to get the word out. It wasn't pretty; I was back in the old mentality of an out of control stutterer. I set about shooting down the challenging word, and was consciously happy I had done that, by practicing saying that particular word over and over in as many similar situations as possible. But that wasn't enough; I was back in the stuttering jungle and was struggling to speak again. I was holding back and back to my old self. I was too self-conscious.

I went on my second speech therapy course in 2002, and got my confidence level and speech back up. I now realised that the fellow participants on the course were in my comfort zone, I had absolutely no fear talking to them. Subsequently, it dawned on me that people who stutter were also in my comfort zone. I had not put people who stutter on a pedestal like I had put the rest of the world. They were at my level. Realising that I was actually comfortable talking to a group of people without stuttering was amazing. In my previous years of speech therapy that thought hadn't crossed my mind. I had attended speech therapy with other stutterers and yet at that time I can't remember having such a thought. I just couldn't speak to anyone.

For the first time in my life I could pick up the phone and talk with such confidence and eloquence. It was eye opening. I even figured out if a fellow stutterer called me the high level of speech would remain. And more excitingly if I had a thought that a phone call was from someone who stuttered I could easily say 'Good afternoon', which had become a challenging phrase. Outstanding Dr Watson! So, in some occasions I would mentally rehearse the possibility that a fellow stutterer was calling me and the speech would be good.

But conversely, if a thought crossed my mind that it was someone important and I didn't want to stutter, I would obligingly stutter right on cue. This was another insight on the journey to freedom.

However, I was ambushed once again, pretty soon after returning from the second course. After many more courses, I realised that my freedom laid on discovering my own path. I was always lucky that I performed well at job interviews, and so I landed my second dream job with the Foreign Office traveling the world and staying in five star hotels.

It was, in one such meeting when working in Washington DC, where I was the team leader, that I was ambushed and held at gunpoint by the stutter. I was right back in the jungle and it would take me a few years to find my way out of this one. I was having chest freezes like a panic attack, the stutter had taken on a life of its own and was a runaway train wreck waiting to happen. The stuttering habit cost me a lot but the one that I will always regret is not taking a risk with a girl. Life is about experiences and the road not taken will always be on my mind.

I was knee high in the stuttering jungle. My speech was so bad that I made my name even shorter, from a two syllable word to one syllable - Ram. That was six years ago. In the intervening years the speech went up and down, and it was when I met my future wife that things started to fall into place. I struggled to say one particular word, which my future wife thought was quaint. That was my first positive experience with a woman who I was interested in. I did date, but that was all. I did go out with women but this was the first time that I met someone who liked me for who I was. And, at that time I was a person who was enjoying travelling and meeting lots of new people. After all, I was living the dream in Buenos Aries, Argentina. The time travelling helped me to develop an inner belief in myself that I would be ok. I had learnt Spanish so was enjoying practicing speaking with everyone, even though I would sometimes struggle saying words.

The last time I was ambushed was in a store. I wanted to attract the attention of the store manager, but I was undecided whether to say 'Excuse me' or call out his name 'George'. In that instant, I hesitated on 'Excuse me.' I use the word hesitated quite deliberately. I did not need to stutter or need to have the label of stutterer any longer. And so, instead of beating myself up with the stuttering broomstick I thought to myself, 'Ah, I stumbled over a word due to not being sure what to say, so forget it and move on. George certainly has!'

Looking back, that was the moment I now realise, "I no longer needed to stutter." I had stumbled over a word. So what! Prime Ministers, Presidents, Kings and Queens stumble over words. Next!

Thought for the Day: "Success is a process, a quality of mind and way of being, an outgoing affirmation of life." Alex Noble

Talking point: Have you ever wondered why you worry so much about your speech? Does it really matter if you stuttered uncontrollably like I did with my boss? In my case, yes it certainly did. I wanted to be able to communicate. Would it matter if I took 1 minute to say what I wanted as long as I was in complete control of the speech process? Well it shouldn't, but I didn't want to sound different. Whenever I made a conscious effort to speak a maximum of 3 words per breath, I could speak without a problem. However I sounded very strange or so I thought. Did I prefer to stutter or to speak in this slow manner? Subconsciously I felt I had to speak faster. Yes I spoke very well and without stuttering when I was speaking in this slow manner but I didn't want to be different. And yet, I was different. All I had to do was open my mouth and the unconscious pattern of stuttering would reveal itself. I had a quandary. What would I would? Well, for the previous 16 years as part of the speech therapy programme I was encouraged to go to support meetings and repeat 3-day fix courses. I had a choice. To return to the herd and be a recovering stutterer or to speak in a conscious controlled purposeful way to become free. Guess which option I went for.

DAY 79: HOLDING BACK

The concept of holding back was new to me. I first heard about it in 2001 when I enrolled on a speech therapy program. The importance of non-avoidance and expanding the comfort zone was preached. I didn't realise the importance of these concepts until much later in my stuttering freedom journey.

I was a card carrying lifetime member of the holding back club. As long as I could remember I would hold back. I wasn't comfortable with putting my head above the parapet so that's how I lead my life. I didn't want to stand out, but the stutter made me stand out. Funny how life makes you do what you don't want to. Everyone knew who I was. I was the stutterer.

Holding back is defined as not doing what needs to be done. As a person who stuttered I had to reinvent myself as a person who was free to express themselves. By avoiding situations and people this not only made sure I would be trapped forever in the stuttering world, it also meant I wasn't living life. Now I know for sure the creator wants to experience life and it experience life through each and every one of us.

To not hold back means I needed to experience an apocalypse every day. The word apocalypse is from the Greek meaning to disclose or reveal. Within my subconscious I had an enormous fear of stuttering. I was trying so hard consciously not to stutter, to avoid stuttering and so consequently I would stutter. By choosing to have an apocalypse moment everyday it sends a message to the subconscious mind that in fact I am proud of the fact I have a stutter and am working on my speech. The more I did what was difficult the easier it became. Practice makes perfect. By experiencing the apocalypse the subconscious mind will eventually see that stuttering isn't something bad or to be avoided.

In my life I held back from a multitude of things. Ranging from not going out to not asking girls out; not asking for a pay rise and staying in a job too long as it was comfortable. My mind was conditioned to hold back. It wasn't the stutter that ruled my life; it was the mindset of holding back that ruled my life. By choosing to express myself openly as a person who stutters and is working on my whole self, the subconscious mind will learn that stuttering serves no purpose and so the stutter will dissipate. In fact, it's ok to stutter and there is nothing wrong with the actual stuttering. It's the meaning I attached to the stuttering that meant something. If I was deaf and didn't hear myself, would I know that I was stuttering?

Thought for the Day: "The only thing holding us back is ourselves." Brad Henry

Talking point: Have you ever examined your thoughts? There are so many thoughts flying round and round and most of them are the same. One insight that I gained was when I wanted to impress someone I would stutter more. The thought I would have is, "This is someone important and I don't want to stutter." Why didn't I want to stutter? Well, at that time I didn't want them to know that I was a stutterer and would try my best to hide it, so consequently I stuttered. When I truly embraced the concept of conscious, controlled purposeful stuttering that was the day I became free.

DAY 80: THE FLUENCY TRAP

For over 30 years my goal was not to stutter and be fluent. I dreamt of speaking normally like everyone else. I dreamt of waking up and not remembering I stuttered. I dreamt of roaring like a lion and speaking my mind without worrying what other people would say. I remember constantly being concerned about what others would think. I spent my whole life listening to the inner worrier.

Since the age of eight all the professors of speech therapy told me not to stutter. Take your time, breathe, slow down, think clearly what you want to say before speaking. This was all good advice, but for me the fallacy of this was the message that stuttering was bad and something to be avoided at all costs. That is where the problem lied. The stuttering itself wasn't a problem. It never was. The stutter was a manifestation of how I was as a being. I wasn't comfortable being me. If no one had pointed out to me I had a big spot on my nose I would have never known or cared. However, like Pinocchio my nose grew and grew. The fear of stuttering when speaking grew and grew as doubts were watered by the imagined limitations of my childhood stuttering mind. At the age of 11, I had a chance to break free by giving a speech in front of the school. I chickened out and 30 years later I went on BBC radio to break free from my imagined limitations.

The stuttering is just the tip of the iceberg. Just as the captain of the titanic who saw the tiny iceberg in the icy ocean waters and commanded, thinking his ship was unsinkable, to plough straight ahead, only to have the iceberg reveal it's underbelly by ripping off ship's starboard, the stutter is just the tiny part that is visible to the outside world. There is a plethora of emotions and memories hiding just below.

The subconscious mind is said to be a million times more powerful than the conscious mind. The speaking process is a subconscious routine. My speaking was a habituated way of producing sounds that I had learnt over a period of time. The repetitions of sounds and words is a normal way of learning to speak. On Kids TV, the phonetic alphabet is taught with the repetition of syllables and then the word. For example A A apple; A is for A A Apple. This is the way that all children learn to speak but in the case of 5 % of children this way of speaking remains till adulthood and beyond.

The repetition of the mantra that stuttering is bad and must be avoided results in the child attending speech therapy thereby learning speech control techniques such as fluency shaping and easy onset. By only treating the tip of the iceberg, none of what is really powering the subconscious routine of the habituated way of speaking is dealt with.

Life is one habit. You wake up at a certain time, brush your teeth in a certain way, have more or less the same breakfast, commute the same way usually at the same time etc. That is usually how your day and your life goes. Unless a spanner hits the works and then all hell breaks loose. The reason is the brain likes predictably. It's primary and secondary function is to protect you and do the least amount of work. In effect your brain wants you to be lazy. It takes a great amount of energy and effort to reprogram yourself.

Consciously breathing and speaking takes effort. That's why your speech is great on courses where you are really making an effort. But you feel totally physically and mentally exhausted. When you go back home and to your workplace, the speech may have improved for the first few days but sooner or later it's goes to pot. That was the story with me for over 16 years of being in speech therapy.

Like anything in life it takes practice for something to become perfect. That's where discipline, dedication, drive, persistence, passion and purpose come in. If you are not committed to making a change then nothing will change. It is in the commitment of creating a new habit, such as reading for 66 days, that will command your subconscious to make the change permanently. Just like riding a bicycle took a few weeks of practise, it's exactly the same with speaking. The habituated way of stuttering when speaking, built up over years and layers of negative conditioning has led you to speaking like the way you do. Once you are committed to the process you are on the way to freedom.

Fluency is a by-product of a life that is not inhibited by the mirrors of the world. As a child your teachers, parents, peers all pointed out there was something wrong with the way you spoke and consequently you tried your best to stop that way of speaking. Over time you began to be fearful of speaking and held back in life. This may have been small things at first, such as telling your classmate the answer to a question in response to your teacher, as you began to be afraid of speaking in a way that was different and had feedback from your peers through their laughter. I still remember to this day when I told my friend the answer to a question in class as I was too afraid to put my hand up. I had become aware that I spoke differently to others and didn't want to be ridiculed.

Laughter is the best medicine but in the case of a stutterer it's the nail in the coffin. Now it's time to work on the inner game and enjoy speaking and conversing with people.

Thought for the Day: "No one knows for sure if you can inherit a stammer, and so I worry that my baby might. It's why I want to work on my speech before he arrives. I don't want him to hear me stammer." Gareth Gates

Talking point: Are you a stutterer and do you have a young child? Do you worry he might pick it up from you? I am a parent of a 2 year old and I am well aware of my thoughts about him stuttering. I also aware that my stutter dissipated at around the time of his birth and I am make sure I speak in a controlled conscious way when around him.

DAY 81: ICEBERG

American therapist Joseph Sheehan first described the stutter as an iceberg. This is to illustrate that most of what occurs in a stutterer are the emotions that are below the surface. The blocking, facial expressions, tics and body moments can all be seen. However there is so much more going on. The feelings and life I led due to the stuttering were the damage caused by the outer physical manifestations of the blocking and sound repetitions. The physical expressions of stuttering didn't matter at all. I wouldn't have realised that I stuttered if no one had labelled me. I wouldn't have cared I stuttered if no one laughed at me. I wouldn't have experienced the life of a stutterer if no one had made me feel different.

Up until the 1970s when Sheehan developed this model, most speech therapists would just treat the stutter. This was indeed the case with me in the 1990s. I had learnt several speech modification techniques but to no avail. The stutter would return within a few weeks or months. There was no long term solution. Looking at the iceberg it shows that about 10 percent is the actually stutter, whereas the rest of the iceberg below the waterline is emotional. So if the stutter is the focus of treatment then only 10% of people will stop stuttering long term. And that has been the case. Treatment for adult stutterers hasn't been very successful. If one, then looks below the waterline at the emotional level of the iceberg, where 90% of the problem exists and treats this instead, a higher level of long term success can be achieved.

Each stutterer has led his life and coupled with the beliefs about himself this has resulted in a lifetime of stuttering. I now propose that stuttering is a habit and like any habit it can be transformed. By working on the whole self, along with the emotional and psychological facets, the stuttering can dissipate and it certainly has in my case.

Research has shown that up to 70 percent of people who stutter may have an inherited predisposition towards stuttering. Yairi and Ambrose Early Childhood Stuttering. Austin: Pro-Ed; 2005. In my family I have a cousin and his son who stutter, so I would have to concur that in the DNA of my family, there is more than a slight possibility of a predisposition to stuttering.

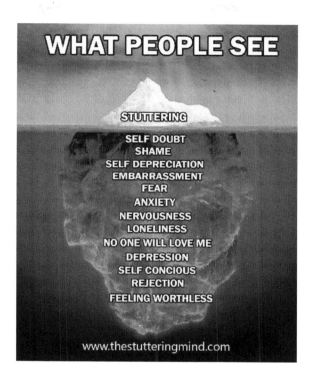

As a person who stutters, it was always that part I didn't want the world to know. I didn't want people to see that I stuttered. I didn't want to be laughed at or looked down. I always wanted to be in the cool gang but was on the outside looking in.

secret code: 918273645

Thought for the Day: "The mind is like an iceberg, it floats with one-seventh of its bulk above water." Sigmund Freud.

Talking point: Why do you think the majority of speech therapy treatments focus on the physical aspects of stuttering?

DAY 82: CLASSROOM

I s life merely an illusion, something that is not what is appears to be? The five senses all provide data for the brain to process what is around it, but what is really going on underneath the drama called life? Why is that when we have a nightmare, we wake up and realise it was just a dream and forgot about it? Could dreams actually provide us with a clue, that in reality life is also a dream; and when we leave this physical body we actually wake up to the truth that we are part of God and we were never actually separate?

Can you actually believe what you see? The electromagnetic spectrum is all the wavelengths of light. However, we can only see visible light. Bees and butterflies see ultraviolet light that enables them to seek out the nectar in flowers. Snakes can sense infrared thermal radiation which helps them go hunting at night. Radio waves, microwaves, x-rays are bouncing around us. Since we don't actually see them, it doesn't mean they don't exist. It's just the waves have been filtered out by our eyes. That brings up a question. What else has been filtered by our eyes and our brains? What is reality? Some people are clairvoyant and others clairaudient. Is it simply, they are tuned into another frequency, so they see a fuller picture?

Just suppose we are immortal beings, incarnating from time to time to experience the illusion of being human. This illusion meant, I was in the pain I had as a stutterer and was lost in my own world of doubt, self- hate and misery. Years of stuttering meant I was holding back from life and the result, I was in my shell. What if, there was a point to this stuttering? It showed me the path to introspection of the inner world, rather than feed the illusion of the outer world. Is there any possibility that I created the experience of being a stutterer? What possible benefits did I get being a stutterer? Granted I am a good listener, patient, empathic and kind. Is it possible, I may have not had these traits had it not been for a stutter?

I had the victim mentality for the longest time and always thought why me? Why did I stutter? I am now at the point of thinking what if there was a purpose for the stutter and my role was to overcome it? If indeed, the inner world is a reflection of the outer world and it is with our thoughts that we create reality and not in fact that life just happens, then I am of the belief that there is something greater going on rather than us as humans just spinning our wheels.

Robert Schwartz, author of Your Souls Plan and Your Souls Gift, used to be in the corporate world employed as a marketing consultant had a career crisis. He went to see a psychic medium. She stared to channel non-physical beings, spirit guides, who told him he had planned his life including his challenges before he was born. They were able to tell him specifically what his challenges had been and were able to explain why he wanted to have those very difficult experiences and this rocked his world. For the next days and weeks after that session with the medium he thought about this perspective constantly. The effect it had on him was it allowed him to review the course of his life and for the first time in many instances, see a deeper meaning or deeper purpose to the challenging things that happened.

Shortly thereafter, he had what is to this day was the single most profound spiritual experience he had ever had. Schwartz shares, "I was doing nothing more than walking down the sidewalk one day, when I was overcome by this feeling of overwhelming, unconditional love for every person I saw and when I say unconditional love in this context drama, I don't mean the kind of love somebody might feel for a parent or a child. This was truly an experience of divine love, it was a transcendent experience. Everywhere I looked, every time I saw another person, I felt pure, divine, unconditional love for them and as this was happening, I understood intuitively what it meant, which was, it was my soul saying to me this love is who you really are, this is your true nature and I believe that my soul gifted me with that experience that day because later on when I went on the write your souls plan and your souls gift, and looked at many, many, many people pre-birth plans. Every single plan I looked at, without exception was always based on great wisdom and unconditional love. I think, if I had not had that experience of myself, my soul, as unconditional love as I was walking down the street that day, I would still have found that same result in my research for the books but they would always have been doubt there, I would always wonder, is this really true? Are all life plans based unconditional love? Well I know it to be true, because that was my experience that day."

He is now a certified hypnotherapist who offers spiritual guidance and hypnotherapeutic regressions to help people understand their life plan. To the question of there being only one life plan or backup plans, Schwartz answers, "Well there's a plan A but there's also plan B, C, D, E, F and on and on. What you could call back-up plans and there is so many of those if it's really beyond the comprehension of the human mind. The reason you have all of these back-up plans is that your soul knows that you have free-will, your soul wants you to have free-will because that's what makes the Earth experience truly meaningful and your soul knows that by making free-willed decisions, you aren't always going make the most loving choice or the most high vibrational choice and so you'll end up on what could be called plan B or C or D, but that's not a bad thing, that's understood to be the Earth experience."

The best way to find out what your life plan is to do a lives soul regression, which is a form of hypnosis in which you start off by going through certain mental, physical relaxation exercises, then the hypnotist guides the client into a past life, Schwartz describes it saying, "it's almost always the past life that had a big impact on the plan for the current lifetime. Then the client's consciousness transitions from their past life back home to the other side, so to speak, most people at that point are greeted by one of their spirit guides, you talk to your guide briefly about why you were shown that particular past life and how it affected the plan for the current lifetime and then we ask your guide to take you to the council of elders; which consist of the very wise, loving and highly evolved beings who oversee reincarnation on Earth and they know everything about you, everything about the plan for your current lifetime, everything about every past life you've ever lived. If you get in front of the council of elders, that is potentially a life changing experience because they can answer any question you put to them, why did you plan certain challenges, why did you plan certain relationships, what did you hope to learn, how are you doing in terms of learning the lessons, how could you do better and people will come out of the between lives soul regression and they'll say things like, "the council answered every question I have about my life, I don't have any more questions about my life now." So, again, potentially transformative experience."

Under hypnosis your consciousness is in two places at once. Schwartz explains, "so part of your consciousness goes into the past life and then to the between lives state to talk to the council but at the same time, another part of the consciousness stays in the room where you're doing the session. So, that part of your consciousness is fully aware all times who you are, where you are, who I am and what we're doing together."

In relation to the stuttering and suffering I experienced Schwartz says, "I would say that almost certainly, it was something that you chose before you were born. The more significant a challenge is in somebody's life, the more likely it is that they chose it before they were born. Stuttering was significant enough in your life that you're now talking to me about the significance of stuttering, so given its importance in your life, I would say almost certainly you planned it before you were born. Now as to why you would've done that, there are number of possible reasons, when I researched people's pre-birth plans, one of the things that I did was by working with mediums and channels, I was able to listen to the conversations that had taken place in the pre-birth planning sessions. The mediums were able to access this information through what is called the Akashic record, which is the complete non-physical record of everything relevant to the Earth plain including the pre-birth planning and in listening to many, many pre-birth planning sessions, I noticed that when souls were planning big challenges like stuttering, a lot of the conversation in the pre-birth planning session revolved around the souls desire to cultivate and then express while in body certain qualities that are important to the soul and I gave these qualities the name, divine virtues."

Explaining that I most certainly had planned the stuttering experience to cultivate certain qualities Schwartz says, "my guess would be, that when you planned stuttering, you had a desire to cultivate certain qualities that you hoped would come from the experience of stuttering, as to specifically which one's it is, I wouldn't know that unless we talk to the council in a between lives regression but we can speculate, for example, self-love, is one of the divine virtues. That is something that could grow out of the experience of stuttering depending upon how you respond to the stuttering. So you can see that it might at first present a challenge, you might judge yourself, condemn yourself in some way for having the stuttering and then hopefully over a period of time, you come to see that this is really not to any significance that you are in fact a beautiful divine, sacred, eternal soul and when your identity shifts like that, from personality to soul and you see the beauty of yourself as a soul, that engender feelings of self-love. You can also imagine that patience, for example could come out of the experience of stuttering. You would need to be patience with yourself in order to have as happier life as possible and so as you're going through the experience of coping with the stuttering, hopefully, you can cultivate greater patience in the way you treated yourself and there are number of other virtues that I think could come out of it, things like, compassion, reverence for life, trust and number of others that could come from that."

One of the best ways to come into an understanding of realising you are part of the divine and are here to learn lessons is through prayer and meditation. It's been said that prayer is talking with God or talking with the universe and that meditation is listening to God or listening to the universe. Schwartz explains, "I think prayer and meditation for most people are two of the most important and most powerful tools you have at your disposal. So, for example you could pray to God or whatever your concept of a divine entity is and say, "I would like to understand my divinity, I would like to know myself as an eternal soul, an eternal being, how might do that?" and then you open yourself up to the guidance of the universe and just follow the ques that come to you intuitively."

Schwartz then explains, "Meditation works very much the same way, at the beginning of a meditation, pose one question to your guides, to God or a spiritual figure of significance to you. It might be, "why do I stutter?" or "did I planned stuttering before I was born?" and then in the meditation, just allow your mind to get as quiet as it can be. Thoughts will arise, don't engage with them, just witness them floating gently by like clouds on the horizon and it's not so much that you're going to hear your guides or another non-physical being speak to you in the meditation, although that could happen but it gives your spiritual team the opportunity to plant seeds that germinate sometimes down the road and so days or weeks or months later, you'll just start to come into insights into the spiritual significance of the stuttering and you won't be able to trace back that these insights started in the meditation weeks or months ago, and that's okay your guides don't need you to give credit to them but it will in fact be the case that the seed were planted and they arrived or germinated weeks later as insights, as knowing about the spiritual purpose of meaning of the stuttering."

The key is to do prayer or meditation on a regular basis so that you have time for the spirit guides or God, the divine, to implant ideas into your human mind. Expanding on this Schwartz says, "I think another thing people can do to come into a sense of how they are souls and the stuttering has spiritual meaning is to look for synchronicity, things that appear to be coincidental but really are not. So in another words when you start asking spirit, why do I stutter, what is it's spiritual purpose, what is its spiritual meaning, what can I learn from it, did I plan it, when you start asking questions like that of the universe, the universe often responds through synchronicities. For example, you're driving down the highway one day and you see a billboard with an ad on it, but the way the ad is worded, somehow it answers one of those questions that you were asking or you turn on the radio and the lyrics of the song at that moment have some kind of message for you that answers your questions. Spirit often communicates with us through those kinds of synchronicity, so I would encourage people to be on the lookout for those."

Thought for the Day: "Learn from yesterday, live for today, hope for tomorrow. The important thing is not to stop questioning." Albert Einstein

Talking point: Are you able to explore the possibility that you planned to experience the stuttering? Can you see that it has helped developed self-love, compassion, patience and other virtues?

DAY 83: PROOF OF HEAVEN

M ainstream media has convinced us that there is a heaven and hell and no return. One of the largest areas of proofs that we are in fact spiritual beings having a human experience are the many reports that have come from people who have had near death experiences. Explaining Schwartz says, "There are many books that have been written by NDE experiencers and they report consistently that the other side, our spiritual home is a realm of great love and light and peace and joy. They report they were embraced with unconditional love and complete non-judgement during the time they were back home on the other side before they return to their bodies. There is a huge volume NDE literature, that was actually where I first started to learn about spirituality."

Schwartz shared he started asking spiritual questions of the universe in his 30's and the near death experience literature is what he was guided to read about and he thinks the reason it occurred in that order is that if he had the experience of unconditional love first, he wouldn't have had any framework in which to integrate it but having read the NDE literature first, it gave him that framework. So, when it happened he was able to incorporate it into his life much more easily.

Dr. Eben Alexander is a neurosurgeon, who in 2008, contacted a rare form of meningitis, which meant his neo-cortex was completely destroyed and was in a coma for 7 days. When he woke up, he was a changed man. As a neurosurgeon and a man of science, he didn't have much time for God. He has since written three books, Proof of Heaven, Map of Heaven, and his latest book is called Living in a Mindful Universe. His account of the near death experience has convinced me that life is much more than we can could possibly imagine and helped me further release all the fears I had about speaking.

Dr Alexander first shared how he spent the first 54 years of his life honing a very conventional scientific world view. He worked in neurosurgery, just as his father had done. He thought he had some idea of how brain, mind, and consciousness work. Explaining he says, "that was a conventional view that basically supported the notions of "physical-ism," that is the idea that the only stuff that exists in the universe is physical stuff, and therefore we must explain all of the emergent reality just based on the natural workings and laws governing the interactions of that physical stuff. And, of course, that kind of thinking implies that the brain creates consciousness and that our existence is nothing more than birth to death. It also implies in our modern thinking that we can only know things through the can of our physical senses— through our eyes, and ears, and that kind of thing."

Explaining how everything was turned up on its head during his meningitis episode and how it was a tremendous gift in many ways as it was a perfect model for human death Dr Alexander shares, " My doctors knew when I was first brought into the emergency room, seizing and in coma, that I was extremely ill. They rapidly diagnosed me with a Gram-negative bacterium meningitis. That's about the worst kind of bacterium meningitis you can have. They put me on a ventilator, on three powerful intravenous antibiotics, and I ended up on the medical ICU where I spent the next week languishing in deep coma."

Adding he says, "Now, important to point that the journey I witnessed is one that absolutely involved complete amnesia for the life of Eben Alexander before coma. I had no words, no language, no personal memories of Eben Alexander's life, no personal memories of ever being human or on this Earth. "

He describes his journey into the unknown saying, "I really started with a very empty slate, and that's how it all was with my earliest memories in coma beginning in what I called the earthworm eye view— a very primitive coarse, unresponsive realm, it was like being dirty jello, and I remember this strong sensation of roots, of blood vessels that were all around me. I had no body awareness at all during any part of it. And like I said, no words, language, or any kind of religious or scientific concepts from my life before. It really was an empty slate of discovery. "

Continuing to describe the wondrous journey he shares, "Now, although that earthworm eye view seems to be, the way the universe was, it was the only thing I'd ever known, given my amnesia for everything else. It seemed to last for eons, for a very long time. But in fact, I think that's just because I had no memory formation deep in the middle of that state, and I was rescued. There came a slowly spinning, very pure white light that had fine, silvery, and golden tendrils off of it, and it came towards me, package with a beautiful musical melody served as a portal."

Dr Alexander then explains, "It opened like a rip in the fabric of that ugly earthworm eye view realm and led up into this brilliant alter-real valley that I call in my writings 'the gateway valley.' And that valley was really, I often likened to Plato's World of Forms. It was a world of ideals; there was no sign of any kind of death or decay. Everything was in kind of its perfect state. I remember seeing lush plant life everywhere. This incredible burgeoning kind of jungle of life with flowers and blossoms, buds on trees. Everything blooming and blossoming in full of force, very rich not only visual but tactile memories of what that is. An important part of knowing in these realms especially given that I had no body awareness at all is that we often know through identification, that's why describing these journeys is so difficult. They're often labeled as ineffable, you know, beyond words, and that's because in those realms we're not seeing with the eyes or hearing with the ears. At times we're becoming entire slates of these scenes as part of our education in knowing through this identification process. And so, in that beautiful valley, I could see thousands of beings down below us that in my early writings I called souls between lives, lots of dancing, joy, and merriment. I remember seeing children playing and dogs jumping, just this incredible festivity, and it was all being fueled because up above, there's kind of Earthly but perfect, ideal, Earthly setting in the valley below me where these swooping orbs of angelic choirs—pure, golden, spiritual beings leaving sparkling, golden trails against the blue-black velvety sky. And every bit of that alter-real valley was lit by the light of these bellowing clouds of pure color. I mean, it was just an extraordinary scene that the words pale compared to the reality of it."

Describing this lovely valley while being a speck of awareness on a butterfly wing he shares, "There were millions of other butterflies. They were all looping and spiraling and swarming in these vast formations over this meadow that contained all those souls dancing down below. And I remember witnessing these sparkling waterfalls, the pools, and all of that lovely scenery going on. And I wasn't witnessing it alone because beside me on this butterfly wing was a beautiful girl, a guardian angel as I came to call her. And her message to me was telepathic. She never had to say a word. She was dressed in the very, in the same, very simple peasant garb that I described all those souls down in the valley below us who were dancing, that they were all dressed the same way—bright colors of very exciting but very simple clothing. I mean, it was really remarkable in that sense, and her message to me I believe is the central part of the message. I would say I came back to share over a long period of time and that's the message that I first shared in Proof of Heaven. But that message was, "You are deeply loved and cherished forever. You have nothing to fear. You will be taken care of." And as I put it in Proof of Heaven, there was another part of that message which is, "You can do no wrong," which I wish I had amplified a little bit where is appears in the book because people get the wrong idea. They think you can do anything you want; it doesn't matter. Well, in fact, what I found on this journey is every action we make, in fact every thought we have is crucial. It is recorded by this universe, and when we leave this physical body, we have to go through a life review."

Explaining that this life review is as real as it can be and is not a new age concept but in fact something that was first described at least 2400 years ago by Plato when he wrote about the near-death experience about of the Armenian soldier, Er, Dr Alexander says, "basically our life flashes before our eyes which really means that any residual lessons from life, and that especially is important to note if we've been busy handing out pain or suffering to others and have some amends still to be made, we will feel that during that life review, and that's why it's best - I think the deepest lesson of all NDEs and all these spiritual journeys is to emphasize the importance of the Golden Rule that we should treat others as we would like to be treated because a very concrete example of bearing the brunt of any hardships that we hand out to people is that life review. In fact, I would say the life review replaces for me the concept of hell, of any kind of eternal damnation because you have to reap what you sow. You have to go through that life review as kind of like a corrective mechanism, and although one could almost say that this corrective effort is simply a balance, so that you feel the effect of your decisions on others and that includes all of the good and loving, compassionate, kindness that you handed out in this world. You feel that, too, in that life review."

Explaining further he says, "But it all is balanced in the light of that love, of that divine presence, what you might call God force, that incredibly strong sense of love and comfort that's so many "near-death experiencers" bring back into this world. You know, it's so strong that they can go to the rest of their lives, maybe 50 years or more, without worrying about death because they'll realise that death is not the end. It's actually a rejoining with Higher Soul, reuniting with souls of departed loved ones, and the brilliant, beautiful, comforting light of that infinitely loving source that God force at the core of all conscious awareness."

He shares how that gateway valley was only a stepping stone and even though he had that beautiful girl there to guide him, he says he remembers, feeling he had a sensation of a soft, summer breeze that blew through and it was his first, really kind of re-awakening to the presence from that divine God force that actually goes beyond any possible naming.

Thought for the Day: "As a neurosurgeon, I did not believe in the phenomenon of near-death experiences." Eben Alexander

Talking point: The Day of Judgement as told in the Bible is now shown to be the Life Review. If indeed we are part of the One mind, then it us who will be doing the judging. Can you explore the possibility that it is you who will be doing the judging?

DAY 84: BACK TO EARTH

When Dr Alexander came back to this world he felt the word God was a purely little human word that didn't remotely do justice to the power and unification of that infinitely loving force and he defaulted to calling "Om" because that was the sound that he remembered from that journey.

When people would ask him about the origin of that word 'Om' he explains, "when I was in that core realm, in the highest realm where I'd seen all of space and time collapsing down, even all when I call deep time, which is in a higher ordering of the events and souls and their incarnations, an evolution of consciousness even that deep time of the spiritual realm collapsing down until I was in the core - infinite and inky blackness that filled to overflowing with the unconditionally loving force of that divine presence, that Om of force."

In the weeks and months that followed, he came to realise the force is what we call in our Earthly forms as God, or Allah, or Brahman, or Vishnu, Jehovah, Yahweh, Great Spirit. Explaining he says, "I don't care what the words are. In fact, the words and the religious orthodox in their linguistic frameworks lead us away from the experiencing and the knowing of that force at the very core of our conscious awareness."

Sharing how he thinks that in many ways the modern religious orthodoxies leads us away from a notion of oneness and connection with that God force which he says, "is a real travesty because religion should be a way of refining our relationship to the spiritual, to the fundamental essence of the causative forces in this universe that bind us all together through that love. And that core realm, I saw all of that very clearly, was presented in ways through identification that go far beyond our capacity to use human language to describe, and that's why so much of my work these days involves returning to those realms."

Continuing his story of the epic journey into the realms of consciousness he shares, "Now, it turns out that in my NDE, I would cycle. I would get to that sanctum - that core realm outside of all the infinity, space, time, eternity. And then I would tumble back down to that very primitive coarse, unresponsive earthworm's eye view where everything began. But the good news is by remembering the musical notes of the melody, which were kind of buried into my memory. This beautiful musical progression— a very simple and yet kind of perfect melody—I was able to conjure up that spinning melody yet again and again several times I would do that, when I would find myself back in that earthworm eye view. By remembering the musical notes, the melody of that portal would come to me again, expand like a rip in the fabric of that coarse unresponsive earthworm eye view realm and lead back into that gateway valley. Again, I was always welcomed by that beautiful girl on the butterfly wing with her very affirming and comforting message, and then that would hasten my journey up through those angelic choirs which provided yet another musical portal."

Explaining how the music he heard is not that kind of music that is limited by the physics of our four-dimensional space-time and any kind of music you would hear in this material realm, Dr Alexander shares, "That kind of music goes far beyond; it's kind of the idealized form of music that's where the great composers would achieve their greatest creative inspirations is in that very realm. That's where they would get this kind of idea. But that's why it's so important to develop a meditative practice. I would say that as sentient beings, we all have the power to come to know this truths and develop this relationship with the Higher Soul and with that primordial mind. We simply have to go within consciousness to explore that, and when you realise physical brain is not creating consciousness, it's more of a reducing value or filter that allows primordial consciousness in, then we can all begin to harvest the benefits of going within which is basically our way of getting out to this universe. "

Concluding his coma journey, he shares, he was told in that core realm every time he entered it, not in words but in conceptional flow, "You're not here to stay we will teach you many things but you'll be going back." Dr Alexander even came to believe that going back meant going back to that earthworm's eye view because he noticed that he would tumble back down to that, and then it could just conjure up through memory of the musical melody, that beautiful portal, that light that served as a portal into the higher realms. But as they were telling him in the core with each visit, "You're not here to stay." And finally, there came a time in my journey, where recovering those musical notes no longer worked to conjure up that beautiful portal."

Sharing how he was feeling at that point he explains, "To say I was sad would be a vast understatement. I think if you could imagine monsoon rains throughout all of eternity you might picture my emotional state. But I also knew at that point even though I had been apparently banned from going back into these highest realms in the spiritual, I knew that I could trust that I would be taken care of. I saw thousands of beings going off around me in these vast arcs into the darkness with heads bowed, many with murmuring of sounds coming up from them, with their hands in front of them. I realised that this was an incredible sense of prayer that all these beings were just trying to comfort me even though I was back in that earthworm eye view kind of murkiness."

Sensing he felt tremendous love and comfort just like he had witnessed in those perfect realms of the gateway valley in the core he felt that was a beautiful gift showing a linkage between the earthworm view and the core. He had no idea what he was headed back to, and it was at that point that he saw six faces that would kind of bubble up out of the muck. They were faces of his family.

Explaining how his doctors had perfect evidence from his neurologic exams, specifically from the CT and MRI scans that his neo-cortex was severely damaged, Dr Alexander says, "I could not have had the capacity to even manufacture a hallucination, or a dream, or a drug-effect because all of that would entail, according to modern neuroscience, that at least some part of the neo-cortex still be working."

Upon waking up in ICU he would have no language or recognition of loved ones at his bed side proving how badly his neo-cortex was damaged, Dr Alexander shares, "I had no idea who these family members were. But words and language came back very quickly, literally over the first hours and days of my waking up from coma. Childhood memories came back over a few weeks. All of my semantic knowledge, everything I'd gained through 54 years of life about cosmology, physics, chemistry, biology, neuroscience, neurosurgery, every bit of that came back within about eight weeks. And in fact, memories and conversations I had with my close family over the next few years prove that in fact that memories that had returned to me by eight weeks were more complete than the memories I've harbored before coma, and this is a point we make in our book in Living in a Mindful Universe about how one of the biggest nails in the coffin of a neuroscientific reductive materialism, you know, brain creates consciousness, is the fact that it does not appear that memories are stored in the brain at all. We go through the evidence from this in the book, but that absolutely wrecks that kind of the "Physical-ist" notion of brain creates consciousness and that, you know, the physical is all that exists, when you really cannot put consciousness or memory as having a permanent resonance in the brain itself."

The experience of being in a coma flipped everything upside down for Dr Alexander. He shares, "I realised early on that to have any notion of where this is all going and understanding of it, I have to reject everything that I had assumed to be true, in those first 54 years of going by the scientific world view. What I've come to realise, beautifully is there are many scientists who have been studying non-local consciousness for decades if not more than a century, and so many people are on the same pathway, but what it does is it does a complete flip."

Explaining how his view now takes the lead from quantum physics, Dr Alexander says, "We are all essentially one with the universe, and the sense of self, the sense of here and now in many ways are a fiction that is constructed by our brain really on this side of the veil, and so I've come to see the unity of all souls, how we're all on this together, we're all essentially manifesting the dreams of the one mind of that God consciousness, and that's why it became very clear that all the ills of this world can be handled by appreciating our sense of oneness, of connection that we're sharing the one mind that this is deeply in the kind of determination of the natural order of things through scientific investigations and through all the manner of human experience. So, it truly just an absolute reshuffling and kind of solidification of notions of oneness, of the power of love to heal, how we are all on this together, how we come back to multiple incarnations as far as evolution of all consciousness."

Thought for the Day: "My whole belief system is that our paths are drawn for us. I believe in reincarnation. I believe we're here to learn and grow. We choose how we come into this life based on what it is we have to learn. Some people have harder lessons than others." Gillian Anderson

Talking point: What is your concept of God? Is it a bearded old man sitting somewhere judging you? Or is it in fact a kind and loving force that resides deep within each and every one of us?

DAY 85: KNOW THYSELF

For someone who has lost their way in life through the struggles of stuttering, Dr Alexander's answer would be to "Know thyself." These two words lie over the entrance of the Temple at the Oracle of Delphi in Greece. Explaining further he says, "And as one comes to realise that thy self, your consciousness is actually the one mind that we share every bit of that, that your conscious awareness at its very deepest level, is the original creative source of the entire universe. Then we can realise that knowing thyself has tremendous power and what that involves is going within."

Sharing how before the coma he would tend to identify with the thoughts in his head he says, "I would tend to identify with that linguistic region in the brain, which I could promise you there are two of them - Wernicke's area – the part that receives speech and Broca's area - the part that produces speech. Here in the dominant frontal for Broca, temporal for Wernicke. And those two regions basically kind of pretend to hijack the entire consciousness in the human being."

Describing how he loves the way Michael Singer puts it in his book The Untethered Soul where he calls the voice in the head as the "annoying roommate." He stresses, "That's about the most kind of credibility we should give that little voice in the head. This is not about a rational logical thinking your way to answers. It's about developing the relationship, the origin of consciousness itself of your Higher Soul and with that primordial mind and to do that involves going within."

Explaining how he has meditated for an hour or two a day for the last eight years by trying to quiet that little voice in the head. Usually done by a form of centering prayer or focusing on the breath. For those who have trouble quieting that little voice of anxiety, the monkey mind chattering away, he recommends the tool that he uses and loves very much which is Sacred Acoustics. Developed by Karen Newell and her business partner Kevin Kossi, Dr Alexander shares, "the bottom line is by going within, by realising we are not slaved to our ego and all of its demands, but in fact that each and everyone of us has a higher purpose that we can discover by going within, by coming to recover love for ourselves because my journey showed me more

85

than anything that the vast majority of the world's problems are not because that I don't love my neighbor enough or love my enemy enough, it is that I don't love myself, and by that I mean recovering the incredible power and kind of sacred divinity of that essence of self that has lived many lives. My Higher Soul that is united with many other souls and my soul group as part of this evolutionary process. But when we come into these incarnations, we voluntarily give up some of that knowledge."

Dr Alexander then shares that when we incarnate on this physical plane we have temporally forgotten the power we have. He put it this way saying, "forgetfulness that is part of the package but that's so we are more tending to buy into this kind of one incarnation, it gives us the skin in the game to have that emotional buy-in and power to the journey to feel all the love but also to feel the pain of loss of those things we love, and those people in relationships, and animals, and every bit of what we come to appreciate in these incarnations. But by going within, we can gain a much grander sense of who we are, why we're here, and where we're heading, and I believe that would be the best advice to those that you mentioned that might have lost their sense of purpose and meaning. I would say that this actually is a major symptom of our predominantly secular and materialist view in modern science that our modern culture has taken to heart, where as in fact those scientists who were at the leading edges of work on the nature of consciousness itself are coming to agree that it appears that we really are spiritual beings living in a spiritual universe, and that the entirety of the material or physical universe is simply a projection out of consciousness. We can gain far grander power, in terms of true freewill over controlling our destiny as we come to develop this relationship that primordial mind and our higher soul through meditation."

The concept of fear is one of the important lessons according to Dr Alexander. He says, "I've come to realise from my journey that I should be able in most situations to come up with the notion that "All is well." What that really means is taking a broad enough perspective of my situation, and that again is rising above Eben Alexander's ego and what that ego maybe demanding and wanting in those situations. But that trying to take that higher view, reuniting with Higher Soul in meditation, that is really about developing that connection so as much as, you know, reading the books, watching the DVDs, going to the lectures, talking with other people about these concepts is very important for setting kind of a cognitive framework or structure. Ultimately, the answers lie within us all. And to gain any true knowledge demands personal experience and that's why I believe it's so important to put meditation front and center in terms of these efforts we have to get closer to any kind of underlying truth."

It's about very gentry trying to put the little monkey mind into timeout. The important thing to remember is you are not thinking your way to these answers. It's not using that rational, logical, linguistic voice in the head. That's not how this works, and it involves a tremendous amount of trust in the universe.

The key concepts in meditation is gratitude which as Dr Alexander explains, "is very crucial to setting the energy level for this kind of understanding growth, the notion of "All is well". It is really one of expressing gratitude, and then trust that the universe will offer up what is necessary, and so I make use of my linguistic brain to state a little intention, make a request at the start of a meditation, but then that linguistic voice goes into timeout, and I've learned to then allow the universe to offer me up what I need to know." A stated intention might be something like, "what do I need to know now?" And with any luck a response will be forthcoming.

"Time flow is a fiction derived on this side of the veil through the workings of the brain," says Dr Alexander. Explaining that, "It's like a staged setting that Hollywood might use for filming a Western out on a desert, you know, where the saloons and the general stores have a facade but there's nothing real behind them. This material world is very much like that, where it's all kind of setup because this staged setting that has this kind of pondering, plodding along of past, the present, the future time and yet the thing about time, it's so fascinating when you look at it from a physics standpoint, it's not understood at all. In fact, time flow in our macro world, that is the world of human beings and big objects, bigger than molecules, is only determined."

Explaining how the arrow of time is only determined by the second law of thermodynamics, which is a statistical law governing the behavior of the large amount of particles like atoms, molecules, Dr Alexander says, "But at their level, that kind of atomic and subatomic level, it's not anywhere near as clear-cut. Time seems to move in the loops. In fact, there are only seems to be an eternal present. Past and future don't have any existence in reality and when you get right down into it, look at the way our language works to conspire to kind of give us an idea of time flow and the reality of time, and yet without those kind of linguistic pointers, all we really know is that there is a present and that present is very strong, and even the present is not as much written in the physical realities you'd like to think."

Citing the experimental studies of Daryl Bem, a psychologist from New York City, Bem showed in an article 'Feeling the Future' just how powerfully our concepts of time are wrong, Dr Alexander says, "In fact the human mind seems to either predict or create what's going to happen in an image showing up on a computer screen. His is experimental setup was basically looking at three kinds of images, very, you know, horrific, violent disturbing images or very pleasant, soothing, comforting images or very neutral images. And what he found is that in fact there is a cognitive awareness of sorts that predicts what image is going to come up even before the computer has selected which image to show, and those studies as much as they absolutely violate our notion of common sense and our conventional scientific view of the nature of time. They basically reporting out features of reality that have to do with the fact that mind or consciousness is primordial in the universe, and then all of the physical universe emerges from consciousness itself."

Dr Alexander then shares how meditation offers a beautiful tool for of stepping outside of the illusion of here and now. By going within and transcending that veil that separates us from primordial mind we can reach richer realms of differential time presentation.

Explaining how your belief systems can affect stuttering and how modern medicine is basically built on the idea of the placebo effect, he says," the reality of our freewill as manifested especially to something as profound as placebo effect proves that we live in a mental universe, that mind completely determines patterns and matter, and it's so much of our human beliefs that are self-limited due to the outmoded notion of Physical-ism or the material world saying that the only thing that exist, we forget how much power our mind has over matter. "

He shares the story of Mary C. Neal, an orthopedic surgeon from the American West, who was in a kayaking accident in the late 90's down in Chile where her kayak was jammed in rocks under water for more than 30 minutes. Dr Alexander said, "You don't survive that and come back but she did. She came back after more than 30 minutes underwater with her legs broken, in coma, was resuscitated, and then had a very long and arduous but amazingly profound recovery."

Concluding Dr Alexander says, "So, these stories tell us, that they hint at the power that human beings have to heal themselves and others. When you realise that healing is becoming more whole, more of who we came to this world to be. I would say that such investigations especially with deep meditations and recovering our lives' purpose and the binding force of love that connects us to all fellow beings throughout the universe, but the more we can come to recover that from meditation and through living a life of action that follows the lead that we discover in such meditations it's really the actions that are so important, and I think to many people it's very heartening to see that near-death experiences are important not just because of what they tell us about what happens after we die, but they're especially crucial at guiding the choices we make in living this life, and becoming more of who we are here to be, and that certainly involves becoming more whole, and I promise you that becoming more whole spiritually, that is when I use the word 'spiritual', I'm talking really about the sense of meaning and purpose and also a sense of connection with the one mind. And the more that we can recover that spiritual essence of ourselves, of our past lives, and of our potential future lives, the more we can come to see that, "All is well", and that all the events in this life which includes the hardships and difficulties are there to serve as stepping stones for growth. They are the engines that drive the essence of our souls."

Thought for the Day: "It is easy in the world to live after the world's opinion-it is easy in solitude to live after your own; but the great man is he who, in the midst of the world, keeps with perfect sweetness the independence of solitude." Ralph Waldo Emerson

Talking point: This forgetting of who we really are certainly had me fooled. As a teenager and young adult I could have never believed that I was a part of the One mind and chose to stutter. Can you now imagine the possibility that you are part of the One mind and you chose to stutter?

DAY 86: WHAT DO YOU BELIEVE?

Knowing that the outer world is a reflection of the inner world and the 3-dimensional world we live in is a reflection of the beliefs we hold, the way we can establish what beliefs we hold, is to be very conscious and look closely at what is happening around you. The kind of people, the kind of experiences you draw into your life and particularly in regard to the painful experiences, the sufferings, Schwarts suggests that you, "Ask yourself what must I believe that would energetically draw this into my life? To take a very common example, a lot of people have the belief of feeling that they are unworthy in some way and if you have the feeling of unworthiness or the belief that you are unworthy in some way, you will tend to energetically magnetize into your life, people who treat you as though you are in fact unworthy. Now, this may sound harsh or punitive from the perspective of the personality but I can assure that it's not the universe intention to be either harsh or punitive. The universe is loving and what it's trying to do in its infinite love for you is mirror back to you so that you can find out what lies within your consciousness even if it's at the subconscious level and then bring it into the light of consciousness where you can then set about healing it. So, those people who are treating you as though you are unworthy are mirroring your belief of unworthiness back to you and the universe's hope is that you will become conscious that you have a belief in your own unworthiness and once you know that, you can set about healing it."

To illustrate how free-will works with pre-birth planning Schwartz shares a hypothetical story, "Let's say that there is a soul and I will arbitrarily I'll give the soul the name, Sally. Sally has had a number of past lives in which she made certain plans before coming into body but then when she got here, she differed to the wishes of others, she let other people tell her how to live her life, not an uncommon thing to do. So, when Sally has her life review after those lifetimes and we do have a life review after each life. She sees that she has this tendency to differ to the wishes of others and she resolves to bring it back into body energetically, not for the purpose of expressing it again but rather for the purpose of healing it. Now let's say there is another soul in Sally's soul group, we'll call this soul George, and George has had the opposite tendency, he's had a number of past lives in which he used power inappropriately over others, he tend to dominate others and tell them what to them do. When George has his life review, he sees that he has this tendency and he resolves to bring it back into body energetically, again not for the purpose of expressing it but rather for the purpose of healing it. Because Sally and George are in the same soul group, Sally knows about George's life plan. So she goes to him before either one of them is born, and she said something like, "hey George, I'm bring back into body the tendency to differ to the wishes of other for the purpose of healing it, I see that you are bringing the opposite tendency back into body, the tendency to dominate others also for the purpose of healing it. Why down we agree that when both of us are 30 years old, we will get married and although this is likely to be a turbulent marriage, our hope is that I will learn to stand up for myself and you will learn to respect others." And George said "that is a great plan, let's do it." Now let's say that when Sally is in body and she's 25 years old, she gets a job with an employer whose running rough shod over her, he's treating her with a profound lack of respect, the lack of kindness and let's say she marshals her internal resources and she takes a stand, she said "stop, if you want me to continue working here, you must respect me, you must treat me with kindness." In the moment Sally takes a stand like that, there's a huge increase in her vibration, if she can then sustain that type of vibration until she's 30, now 1 of 2 things will happen, either she and George never meet because by virtue of the law of attraction, her vibration is so much higher than his, they're never drawn together or if they do meet, there is no attraction, there is only 1 date and then nothing comes of it, again law of attraction, their vibrations are too dissimilar so there is no attraction. So, in this hypothetical example, Sally has used her free will to learn her planned lesson, which was to stand up for herself which in turn obviates the need for the planned challenge, the turbulent marriage. Now, someone listening to the stories, is going to think "well what about George?" "Doesn't he still have to learn his lesson?" Yes, he does but he will now call into himself other relationships or other experiences that will give him the opportunity to learn, to respect the wishes of others. So in this hypothetical, you see that intersection between freewill and pre-birth planning."

Explaining how we come into this physical plane in soul groups, Schwartz shares, "A soul group is a collection of souls who are more or less at the same stage of evolution, in other words, the same frequency or vibration. You and the other members of your soul group reincarnate together again and again and again, playing every conceivable role for each other. So, you and the members of your soul group will be mother and daughter, father and son, brother and sister, close friends, bitter enemies perhaps even murderer and the one who is murdered. There is no judgement about any of these roles at the soul level, they all viewed as opportunities for expansion, healing and learning."

Schwartz then shares his definition of the soul and incarnating personality saying, "The soul as what you could call, is a spark of God, and the personality is a spark of the soul, in other words, the personality is a portion of the soul's energy placed into a physical body but your soul is a vast, vast energy field, that spans many dimensions. So, the portion that's in body here in the 3rd dimension is just a portion of that energy field."

Relating to the possibility that there is a Rama out there in a parallel universe that did not stutter at all, Schwartz said, "that is very possible and I would say even likely." He then shares a chapter from Your Souls Gift, about a woman called Beverly who plans a traumatic experience and she plans this for the things that it will teach her. They we worked with a medium who channels Jesus and Schwartz asked him about Beverly. Schwartz then shares, "I asked Jesus, "are there Beverly's in other dimensions who did not experience the trauma?" and he said "yes" and I said, "how many Beverly's are there?" and he said, "about 3 or 4" and I said "well how can it be about, doesn't it have to be a discrete number." And then he draws an analogy he said, "think of this soul as being like the trunk of a tree and the various personalities are like limbs that grow off the tree and certain limbs grow and they mature and then they die and fall off the tree and then they're replaced by young limbs that start to grow in that place on the tree." So he said, "You know personalities are being formed and dissolving constantly based upon the souls desire, the soul is the eternal portion, the trunk of the tree that carries on" and then he explains that the reason you have their parallel selves in other dimensions, is that the soul wants to experience everything."

Explaining further Schwartz shares, "in your case, most likely your soul wants to know what it's like to be Rama, who has stuttering but also to be Rama who does not experience stuttering and there are probably additional Ramas in other parallel dimensions, who are having other kinds of experiences to round out the experience of being Rama. One thing Jesus says as we're talking about this, is that it's really not necessary for people to concern themselves to much with parallel dimensions, your task is basically to focus on why are you here in the 3rd dimension on Earth right now and learn what it is that you came here to learn."

To figure out if we are on the right path of life is to simply tune into your feelings. Schwartz explains, "people who are off the path that they planned before they were born and I'm referring here to plan A. They have feeling of discontent or what you might even call, divine discontent. So they have this vague nagging sense that there's something else they're supposed to be doing here, they don't know quite what it is but they do know, that whatever it is they're doing right now, that isn't it and I had that feeling myself back when I was in the corporate sector, I knew intuitively quite strongly that, that was not what I was supposed to be doing but I didn't know what it was I was supposed to do and it took a little while to figure that out, the session with the medium certainly helped quite a bit, but if you have that feeling of divine discontent, that's not a bad thing, that's your soul gently nudging you to know that there is something else you're here to do and as you go about exploring it, it will become clear what it is."

Thought for the Day: "The future belongs to those who believe in the beauty of their dreams." Eleanor Roosevelt

Talking point: Do you know what your beliefs are? If you look around you, what you see reflects your subconscious beliefs. If you really believe you will be a millionaire like Gary McEwen, founder of Trustatrader.com did, then you will be. If you believe you will always stutter, then you will.

DAY 87: YOU ARE NOT A VICTIM

Schwartz shares what he was told by a respected source when he asked about Hitler, "Believe it or not, his pre-birth plan was to be a great spiritual leader and his soul endowed him with certain gifts that were intended to facilitate that, gifts of oratory, gifts of rhetoric, gifts of charisma, all of those gifts were intended to allow him to become a great spiritual leader but as we have discussed here, we all have free-will. Hitler, as I understand, had a very difficult upbringing and he responded to that by making a free-will choice to go in to opposite direction of his initial pre-birth plan. So, he deviated from his pre-birth plan about as much as anybody could have. Then I asked the same trusted source, where is Hitler now, what became of him, what I was told is that he's back on the other side and is aware of what he did and how wrong it is and he's punishing himself by constantly recreating his own physical death, which apparently was quite painful in his incarnation as Hitler. Now it's important to say here that, he's not being punished by God or by any other being external to him, this is a self-inflicted punishment, but he is loved as unconditionally as all the rest of us are. He's surrounded by guides and angels who are beaming love and light to him, he just can't perceive the love and light, but eventually he will then he'll move into the light, he'll stop recreating his painful death and at that point, presumably, he will be aware that he has quite a bit of karma to balance and will start reincarnating in order to balance it."

With regards to people who are facing hardships on this physical plane Schwartz shares, "souls depending on how old they are, their age as a soul, they want to have certain kinds of experiences when they come to Earth and in particular, the youngest souls who haven't been on Earth very much, they are interested in exploring issues of physical survival, on then physical plain, so they will tend to incarnate in a place like Africa and perhaps experience something like starvation, because they're exploring survival on the physical plain. Then when you get just a little bit older, souls become interested in exploring issues of power. Those souls will tend to incarnate in a place like the United States, which lends itself to exploring issues of power and then you get into mature soul, an old soul, those souls, according to Michael, incarnate in certain regions of US and Canada mainly the Pacific Northwest at cities we would call 'New Agey' like Ashland, Oregon, Arizona, Sedona or Ashville, North Carolina. The mature and older souls are also incarnating in certain countries, the Scandinavian countries, Poland, Switzerland and Michael says that the mature and older souls are interested in exploring issues of relationships, emotions and psychological subjects."

Explaining that physical illness could be a sign that you're off your intended path but it isn't necessarily the case, Schwartz says, "there are other reasons why physical illness can occur. A lot of times it's just in service to others, for example, let's say that somebody wanted before incarnating to have an experience of being a caregiver, maybe they're working on developing patience, unconditional love, compassion and so forth. So if they're going to have to play the role of care giver, someone then has to play the role of receiving the care and somebody might plan an illness in service to the caregiver so that they could have the experience of the caregiving and cultivate virtues like compassion, patience and unconditional love. So, basically if you have an illness and you're trying to decide, does it mean that you're off your path. You can't necessarily assume that's what it means it could have other significance but it could mean that you're not on your highest path. A lot of times also, physical illness will occur when someone is just rushing around in a very mindless manner, trying to franticly accomplish as much as they can, trying to do multiple things at the same time and basically not paying attention to the underlying lessons that they came here to learn. With someone like that, the soul will start by sending very minor physical ailments in a way to slow them down, and if they don't then slow down and start to live in a more conscious manner, then something more serious may happen. You know if you have that pattern in your life of a particular kind of challenge, like an illness coming back around and in particular if it comes back in increasingly intense form each time, that is really something to pay attention to because that's your soul tapping you on the shoulder and trying to get your attention, trying to get you to look at something that you are missing."

Sharing how you can use the law of attraction to do just about anything you would like to do and that law of attraction is one of the main underlying laws of the universe, Schwartz explains, "it basically says that like attracts like, so if you stutter and you would like to change that, the way to do it is to raise your frequency, raise your vibration as much as you can. So you can go about that in the couple of ways, one is, instead of focusing on the stuttering, you can focus on whatever is working in your life and as you feel grateful for the things that are working, your vibration increases and then you draw to yourself by virtue of law of attraction, things of equal frequencies which will be enjoyable experiences. The other way to go about using law of attraction, to work on stuttering would be to look closely at the stuttering itself and identify what good things either are coming out of it or could come out of it and then you change your vibration because instead of viewing it as a problem or as a meaningless form of suffering, you start to view it as a learning opportunity and when you do that, again, your vibration increases and then you draw to yourself things that are equally high vibration."

Explaining the single most important thing that pre-birth planning does for a person, Schwartz says, "is that it pulls them out of victim consciousness, in other words, you come to understand that you are the powerful creator of what you experiencing in your life and when you come into that awareness you realise that you are not a victim, that in fact really nobody is a victim."

Schwartz goes on to share, "victim consciousness is the single, lowest frequency or vibration a human being can be` at and it tends to be self-perpetuating because when you believed yourself to be a victim then you vibrate at the frequency of victim and when you vibrate at the frequency of victim, you are energetically stating to the universe that you are a victim. Well, whatever energetic statement you make to the universe, the universe always responds in the same way, it always responds by saying, "yes, that's right, you are." So if you state energetically to the universe that you are a victim, the universe says, "yes, that's right, you are a victim" and then it brings to you more experiences that seem on the surface to confirm to you that you are in fact, a victim. The way to break out of that negative self-reinforcing cycle is to understand that you planned your challenges before you were born, again, that pulls you out of the frequency of victim, then you no longer vibrate at the frequency of victim, then you no longer state to the universe that you are a victim. So, you magnetize to yourself much more enjoyable experiences."

Explaining how limiting beliefs such as low self-love and lack of worthiness, powerlessness and scarce resources and how the outer world reflects this to us in order to learn lessons Schwartz shares, "it's basically law of attraction, so the way you might think of it is that whatever you believe, you're vibrating at the frequency of those beliefs. It's like when you drop a stone into still water, you drop a stone into a pond and then the vibration, the ripple's expand out in concentric circles, you are always sending energy out away from the physical body in concentric circles and those waves radiate out, very, very far and then they draw back to you experiences that reflect your beliefs and they are at the similar frequency or a similar vibration. So when you're trying to assess what are your beliefs and do any of them needs to change, just look very closely at the kinds of experience, the kinds of people your drawing into your life and then ask yourself, what must I believe if these kinds of experiences and people are coming into my life. Once you got an answer to that question, if it's a false belief, set about changing it in a very conscious manner, tell yourself on a regular basis that, that belief is false, substitute what you know to be a correct belief and as you do that repeatedly and consistently over a long period of time, you'll draw to yourself by virtue of law of attraction more enjoyable more positive experiences and then once you see, the world mirroring back to you your more positive beliefs and then you'll be convinced that those beliefs are actually correct."

Concluding Schwartz shares, "I think the most important thought that I would like to leave is that the Earth as I understand it is not literally the most difficult place to have an incarnation but it is considered one of the most difficult and the simple fact that you are here in body at this time on planet Earth, makes you among the most courageous souls in the universe. There are lot of souls who know there would be great value in incarnating on Earth but they don't actually have the courage to come here but any one reading this did, so I would invite you and encourage you to honor and recognise the great courage you show in coming to planet Earth, only the most courageous, incarnate here."

Thought for the Day: "The height of your accomplishments will equal the depth of your convictions." William F. Scolavino

Talking point: When I was stuttering like a parrot, I could have never imagined the possibility that I actually planned to have a stutter. Now, with the hindsight of stuttering freedom I can quite believe that the stutter served a purpose. What about you?

DAY 88: DREAMS

A dream will always be a dream if no action is taken in moving towards that dream. Defining goals that make up your dream will certainly make the dream a reality. As a person who stutters, for the longest time my dream was to be able to speak without stuttering. I didn't want to show the world that I was 'inferior' and so by hiding the part of me that was ashamed of my whole self I would never be able to speak. However, I also had a dream of being an author and speaker. I had also enjoyed writing. But failing my English exam at school meant I had subconsciously been programmed, "I couldn't write." And yet 4 years later, I retook the English exam and got an A grade. What had changed in the intervening four years? I had gone to university and had learnt how to structure an essay. And so I started my first novel at the age of 22, which I will be completing as soon as I finish "The Stuttering Mind" book series.

The dream of being an author meant I had to get out of the stuttering mindset. I had the mindset of someone who was playing on the sidelines. I was on the substitute bench for most of my life. I was the last one to be picked at school for football teams and this scenario was the case in all areas of life. At a young age I had learnt not to put my head above the parapet in case someone got an axe and chopped it off.

When I was 6 years old, I remember feeling terrified of failing an end of year exam and not going on with my friends to the next class. I have absolutely no idea why I was so afraid, but I also remember seeing my friends enjoying themselves while I was looking on. When I was 13 years old, I was lucky enough to board a real English battleship. However I was close to missing out. I went with my mum and she left me with one of her colleagues. It was symptom of my stuttering mind that I had was always on the sidelines. I was waiting patiently to be called. But no one called me, until the last moment, when someone noticed me and hurried me along to join the rest of the children. This sitting on the sidelines of life would play out numerous times over my lifetime.

I could have sat out again, but this time I made a different choice. I chose to get married and happily my girlfriend at that time agreed. I always had a dream of getting married and having a son. And so it proved to be.

Getting married was one of the most important decisions and looking back from the point of someone who stuttered it proved crucial. Having someone who loves you and wants to be by your side through life's trials and tribulations helps the core beliefs of I am worthy of love. I had developed beliefs that were unhealthy. It's interesting that even some of the most successful of businessman have beliefs that have been created from childhood.

Parental expert Shelly Lefkoe shared with me in Rich Thinking explaining, "Our beliefs stay with us throughout our entire life." She has clients who have doctorates from Harvard University, but are still plagued by a belief that they are stupid because of beliefs they acquired in childhood, when they were between six and eight years old." Having a son is God's gift. The universe blessed me with a son, and seeing my baby son grow has proved to be one of life's teachers.

The dream for me was to be my true self, express my thoughts and feelings without holding back and pursue a life filled with joy, enthusiasm and happiness. To achieve this dream I had several goals:

- Enjoy each and every day and doing work like it was my hobby
- Enjoy meeting and really conversing with people
- Remember the truth we are all 'One' and there is nothing to be afraid of
- Remind myself to really be present and enjoy the moments

Tom Corley and Vishen Lakhiani, shared their dream setting exercises with me. Go to www.richthinking.net/stutteringfreedomdreams to download the template.

Thought for the Day: "A dream doesn't become reality through magic; it takes sweat, determination and hard work." Colin Powell

Talking point: Have you ever thought about what it is you really want to experience in this life? If you haven't, then the dream setting process will most certainly help you.

DAY 89: HABIT

Stuttering was a habit I had for over 30 years. The anxiety, incorrect breathing, incorrect voice productions, feeling of being rushed, fears and negative self-talk over the time period resulted in a poor speaking manner. I would rush to get the words out so as not to stutter. I learnt from my good friend, John Harrison, many years ago at a Neuro-Semantics workshop in London, by doubling the volume of the voice and halving the speed of speaking, it will help you control your speech.

Some people may find it hard to think of stuttering as habit but truth be told it most certainly is. Stuttering is a combination of incorrect habits that has produced this way of speaking. If former US Vice President Joe Biden can overcome stuttering in his 30's why can't you? There is absolutely no difference between the US Vice President and you. The only difference being is whether you believe it's actually possible to become free and start working on your mindset.

Incorrect breathing habits and incorrect speech production has created the stuttering pattern. This is your way of speaking. Whenever I approached a speaking situation I would feel afraid and apprehensive. This fear would cause me to be anxious and stressed. Inevitably stuttering would be the result. It's a subconscious routine.

99% percent of humans speak subconsciously without doubt entering their mind. The lack of discipline, focus and control consciously has led you to the speaking in a way that is out of control.

When you started to learn how to drive a car for the very first time you had to be conscious of where to put your foot on the clutch to change gears in a manual stick shift car. You also needed to be alert to other cars in your vicinity before you set off. It took a tremendous effort and concentration just to do all these things in order to drive. Then after a few weeks you realised you no longer needed to concentrate as much when changing gears. This conscious process was now part of the subconscious. And after a few months while driving you noticed your thoughts are not entirely focused on driving.

Just like driving, your speaking pattern has become a subconsciously routine. Your breath, your heart beat, the way you walk and the way you speak are all run by the subconscious. Imagine you had to tell your heart to beat every second. Or imagine you had to consciously take a breath in each time. Well as a person who stutters that's what you need to do. You will need to consciously learn to breathe again using your upper and lower diaphragms so that you will have a full intake of air in your lungs so as to be able to produce sounds and words. You will need to practise saying the alphabet, just like my two year old son.

In my book Rich Thinking I shared what Allon Khakshori, the former manager of Novak Djokovic told me:

The turning point for Djokovic, said Khakshouri, came after he had been beaten by Federer and Nadal many times at several major events. At some point, he decided that if he were to win, he would need to change his lifestyle, improve his physical fitness and even change his entire surroundings.

Djokovic committed to being the fittest guy in tennis and this transformation paid off towards the end of 2010 when he won the Davis Cup for his home country, Serbia. This, says Khakshouri, was a very emotional win for him. His winning streak continued in 2011 when he won a second Grand Slam title. He is now known as a leading authority in the sport, having shocked many by his transformation and success.

The turning point for Djokovic, convincing him that he needed to work on transformation in his mind, had to do with the fact that he wasn't beating the top two players in the world. This caused him real frustration, and led him to make the decision to really work on himself. The "frustration of not having hit the rooftop," as Khakshouri puts it, "led to him deciding that he would need to completely reinvent himself from the inside out."

You will need to reinvent yourself, just like Novak Djokovic did to win his first grand slam title, in order to become free from the stuttering mind. There is no easy cure to stuttering. You have had this way of speaking for a lifetime and so with time and effort you can and will be free from the stuttering mind. Once the stuttering mind stops the stuttering will stop.

Thought for the Day: "Motivation is what gets you started. Habit is what keeps you going." Jim Ryun

Talking point: How difficult is it for you to accept that stuttering is a habit?

DAY 90: FEARS

Fear is an interesting emotion. It is said that a new born baby only has 2 fears. One is of being dropped and the other is of loud noises. All other fears are learnt and can come up from nothing. Be it, when you are flying in an airplane as a child, suddenly there is turbulence and bang you are afraid of flying. And so it is the case with stuttering. At the age of 8 I was sent to speech therapy jail. I remember two incidents which may have been the trigger to a lifetime of stuttering. A lot of children stumble over words and grow out it, but it was the fear and self-doubt that drew me into stuttering.

I was about 7 years old and in the toilet. I forgot to lock the door and my Uncle walked in and saw me peeing on the seat. He went mental. The other incident was at my primary school. There was a boy who got his mother to speak to me. I guess for some reason the boy wasn't happy with how I was with him, so his mother came up to me one day and man-handled me.

Could these two incidents have triggered me to stutter? Quite likely! As a young child, I wouldn't have been able to process these two incidents, and coupled with my parental and social conditioning of holding back, this would mean I developed a fear of speaking.

I had a belief I would stutter for the rest of my life. Having met a friend who was 18 years older than me who stuttered like a parrot I had no reason to doubt this belief. I was then surrounded by recovering stutterers on a speech therapy programme, so I developed another belief of being a recovering stutterer for the rest of my life. I then lost contact with my friend and most of the recovering stuttering friends. I made friends with people who didn't stutter. I got married and had a son. I now hold the belief of, 'It no longer matters if I stutter.'

Thought for the Day: "If you want to conquer fear don't at sit home and think about it." Dale Carnegie

Talking point: The fear of being judged caused me to become afraid of speaking. Being fearful of authority figures made me stutter uncontrollably. We are our own worst enemy and critic. The day we become 'ok' with the stuttering, is the day the stuttering will dissipate.

DAY 91: THE VOICE

The voice in the head that never shuts up, the 'annoying roommate,' as Michael Singer, describes in his book, The Untethered Soul. This voice was certainly a thorn in my side, constantly talking, constantly worrying and constantly criticising. Have you ever stopped to examine the voice in the head? Is your voice constantly commenting on everything that happens? And when I stuttered, I would replay the same movie in my head over and over again.

As a person who stuttered, I could never really see myself not stuttering. Even though I would dream of the day that the stutter would disappear, I would wake up with the dread of remembering I had a stutter. I was trapped in the mind of a stutterer. I had built up a house of stuttering and the foundations were made of concrete. Despite being on countless speech therapy courses, the stuttering mind persisted. I was surrounded by people who stuttered or were recovering from stuttering. I hadn't met anyone who actually recovered from stuttering. Just like a recovering alcoholic, I thought my life was to attend speech therapy programmes ad-infimum. That was my standard. And so, it was my reality. Once I could actually see myself living a fulfilled life and pursuing my dreams, the stutter dissipated. It was in the quieting of the voice that the realisation of who I really am, was made possible.

Karen Newell, founder of SacredAcoustics.com and is the co-author of a book Living in a Mindful Universe with Dr. Eben Alexander. Ever since she was a child she had burning questions such as, "why are we here?" and "what is my purpose?" Raised as a Methodist in the United States, nobody wanted to hear those questions. They were more interested in how the visible world works, how do the trees grow and why the sun is there? She was suspicious that she wasn't taught the true story of where our humanity's origins came from. So, she went through life looking for these answers turning to texts like the Kabbalah and the Hindu Vedic texts. As she went along reading about all these concepts she realised in order to truly understand it you had to experience the unseen, thus beginning her own practice of meditation to help answer those burning questions.

At first, she felt it was a little intimidating because it was her impression that people who meditate had to have an eastern type of upbringing and have a different point of view. And she thought she would have to assimilate those beliefs in order to meditate. Trying to mediate on her own by watching her breath she found it difficult to settle her mind. As she would go through endless lists and plans in her head while trying to meditate she thought it was a waste of time. Finally by using sound to help settle the mind she was able to meditate on a daily basis for the last 9 years.

Explaining why any time there is a problem in the external world it has to do with something inside, Newell says, "what I've learned is we need to look into what's going on inside, whether it's a past emotional trauma, a belief that we've had from a young age that maybe isn't serving us so well. We kind of attached a lot of different things that we learned as children that maybe they're not very well meaning things that we learned. We may think that we're not good enough or I'm not smart enough, I'm not smart as my neighbour or something. All of these things kind of stick in our minds and it causes problems in the external world and when we can really go inside and start to uncover some of those emotional traumas, some of those not even necessarily traumas, just misunderstandings that we have about our self because of the external world. When we can go inside and start to uncover who we really our and start to become more aligned with that unseen part of ourselves. This really helps us to have greater awareness of what's going on around us, have greater awareness and practice of finding calmness inside and seeing that then the world around us becomes more calm."

In a situation such as stuttering it would be a very similar concept of going within and getting more awareness of that greater part of yourself which will then help you get become more centered, more aligned and the stuttering will fall by the wayside.

For anyone starting out in meditation it is necessary to find techniques that work well for the individual as we are all different. And if one is not working, the best way is to keep trying out different techniques. Newell suggests, "The most basic technique of meditation is to watch your breath, to put your attention on the actual inhale and exhale, just watch yourself inhale and exhale, this is a form of mindfulness."

Mindfulness is the idea that you put all your focus onto whatever activity you're performing in that moment, whether it's walking, studying or just simply being. In the case of meditation, the breath is ever constant, it's ever present, and it's always happening whether you notice or not. Newell says, "It's a very useful handy tool especially when you're first starting, when you're trying to quiet that mind and you noticed the mind wandering, simply return your attention to the inhales and the exhales of your breathing. At first it can seem like I thought, a waste of time but the more time you put in to it, even if it's just 1 minute, 2 minutes or 5 minutes up to 10,

20 minutes a day, you really start to see some progress and there is so much research on meditation and the effect that you will have in your body, really all of us need to be doing this to lower stress, increase our immune system so we're healthier."

Newell shares more of the benefits of meditation saying, "It helps us really to get in to calm states of our parasympathetic nervous system where it is working at its finest. It helps us to lower blood pressure, all kinds of physical things, but it also keeps us calmer, less anxious especially in the world of today that every time you turn on the news it seems that there is another bad thing happening in our world, it's hard to stay calm in a world like this. So, finding that still space inside, really gives us an escape from all of that unrest that seems to be going all around us."

Heart awareness is something that Newell is very much into. Having learnt it through the practice of mediation Newell shared, "I learned about the heart map institute in northern California, who actually study the heart in a scientific way. They have measured an electromagnetic field that comes in and out of our heart and it's in the shape of a Taurus field. It comes out the top of our head around our bodies moving constantly, in all directions. It is centered right here in the heart."

Explaining what is amazing about this electromagnetic field she describes, "it expands and contracts based on our emotional state. Emotions like joy, happiness, or love will create a very large electromagnetic field but emotions like anger, sadness, depressions or grief, those kinds of emotions create a much smaller more constricted electromagnetic field."

Newell adds, "Now what's so fascinating to me about all of this, is this electromagnetic field actually affects the people around us, so we all know these people, at least if you had an office job like I did, one of those 9 to 5 office jobs, where people come in to the office complaining about their commute or something bad that happened that morning, It kind of puts everyone on edge, in a bad mood. Whereas people who come in to the office feeling magnanimous and "oh what a beautiful day" and a big smile on their face, it kind of make us feel calmer. So these studies with heart map, have actually had one person sit across the table from another and the person will perform a technique that they call coherence which is at its basic nature is feeling a sense of gratitude in your heart, simply finding gratitude and feeling it, not just thinking about it. This will create what heart map calls a state of coherence and someone how is coherent, sitting across the table from someone who is not, the other person actually becomes more coherent. Their brain waves and their heart rates variability starts to match the person sitting across from them."

Looking at studies done of couples who sleep together in the same bed it's been found not only their heart rate variability but their brain wave states, seem to synchronize. Newell explains, "So this is a way to becoming aware of your heart actually helps not only yourself but all the people around you and this is what really motivated me because I did not want to have anything in my heart that was potentially putting someone else around me in any kind of distress and so the idea of generating only positive beneficial loving feelings, not just thoughts but feelings in my heart, was a huge task that I undertook and it's not necessarily simple, its sounds very simple but it is not necessarily easy to generate a feeling of gratitude in the heart, and it can take some time to do."

Newell had to rattle through all the things that she had felt grateful for throughout her life. Explaining that for some it might be beautiful nature, a beautiful sunset, it might be the ocean or it might be a person. Newell says, "People are a little tricky because a lot of us will have emotional baggage around a particular person even if it's someone that we love dearly, usually there is some other problem and so it's challenging to think of the person. Babies work too, but they grow up to be teenagers so depending on the stage of your baby that you have in your life, that may or may not work. For me, it was puppies, thinking of puppies."

Remembering to the time when she was six years old and her mother had taken in a stray dog. The dog decided to give birth to puppies underneath her bed. Newell reminisces, "so you can imagine it, age six, what a magical kind of loving moment that was, at least for me maybe not for my mother. So, every situation that presents itself for one person they may feel gratitude and the other may not, so it's very unique kind of feeling and the more I thought of those puppies, the more I recalled that memory, that magical memory of being an innocent child and seeing the beauty of life take form right underneath my bed. When I thought of that, eventually I started to feel this gratitude. So all of us can do this and this is how we become more aware of our heart."

Newell explains, "As you become more aware of what's going on in your heart, you start to pay attention to actually how people around you respond to your heart feeling. You can do this without saying a word, simply feel different feelings in your heart. Feel what it feels like to change the energy inside of yourself and then how people respond around you. This is just something we all have - this heart. All of us have these tools that do this and so becoming more aware of how it affects people around you we can really help ourselves and ultimately our entire world."

Explaining how many of us in our world think about our problems she shares, "we think about who we love, we think about reasons why we behave in ways that we think people will know that they love us but many of us really have been taught to hide our emotions, to stuff our emotions away because it's not necessary acceptable in some societies. I know in some families, mine included, children are taught to be seen and not heard because they are so kind of effusive and emotional all that time and so many of us learned to suppress our emotions and when we have trouble, a particular conflict or trauma in our life. Now these are sweeping generalizations but we are not necessarily taught how to process those emotions. So frequently practicing the feeling of gratitude is beneficial to all of us."

All through my life I never felt worthy of anything. For some reason I had learnt not to put my head above the parapet. At the age of 12 I had learnt to hold back and not stand out from the crowd, perhaps due to the stuttering or due to parental and social conditioning. At my school, I was in the running to be the top student for the year, and would have won a prize. It was the mindset of holding back that led me not to claim an extra 10 points which would have put me in first place. Interestingly 30 years later, I would still think about seemingly insignificant events in my childhood or maybe they were so significant that they shaped my life.

Seemingly innocent comments led my subconscious mind to create my reality. The idea of needing to be perfect and not to stutter made me stutter. The idea of it's not ok to be vulnerable in front of strangers made me stutter.

Describing how the electromagnetic field of the human heart is 60 times bigger than the brain Newell says, "The heart's electromagnetic field is vastly larger than the brain, and I think people who walk around in our world, thinking the brain is everything are people who get PhDs and spend so much time learning. There's nothing wrong with becoming a PhD, but this heart field is actually more powerful than the brain in many ways and we forget about it because we don't attach language to it, we don't attach learning to it. We don't attach positive kind of things that we bring into our world to our heart. Very often we are taught that these feelings of the heart, get in our way and they prevent us, they cause suffering and we want to rise above that suffering but what if that heart, that feeling state is actually an engine that provides us clues to how the world works and what our particular purpose in the world is."

Giving an example of an emotional reaction to something in the external world, Newell shares, "The power of the heart when you have an emotional reaction to something in your external world, this is actually a clue, a signal to you that there is a problem inside that is being reflected by that reaction. So emotions can be used to identify particular triggers for things that are going on in the world and those triggers can be picked through and you need to find out what's beneath those triggers. These are those beliefs, those emotional trauma, those things that we put away and then it gets triggered by those things in our society."

Revealing how Heart map has also found that the heart sends more information to the brain than the brain sends to the heart. Newell shares her take on that saying, "this electromagnetic field is out there not only broadcasting information for others to resonate but it also picking up information and bringing that into our hearts in a form of intuitive feeling and those intuitive feelings, they're coming in naturally and the information that get sent to the brain allows us to then interprets those feelings in some fashion. Usually that interpretation involves assigning words and language which, yes, helps to elucidate the feeling but it also helps to limit the feeling to a particular story and so we want to really be more open to really understanding where our deep, deep feelings come from and this heart energy can really help us get there in a remarkable ways."

Explaining how I thought I stuttered in every single situation and only realising in later years that I stuttered much less with my family, Newell shared how I probably felt safe with my family members saying, "it sounds like a comfort level that when you're with your friends and family, who know you better and who you trust. You have a different kind of connection with them, that is safer and when you get out in the world, it means it's challenging enough for all of us to deal with bosses who ignore us and that is not a good feeling but yes, if you're telling yourself that you are a stutterer and then in those nervous kind of situations, you stutter even more, it is absolutely your reflection."

Adding about how I created my reality with the stories I told myself about being a stutterer, Newell explains, "with those types of stories, they can be self-perpetuating, so as we try to get out of that story of being a stutterer it just seems to get worse until we can really get behind it. So I would say that just those external kind of less safe environment would trigger it to happen even more because it creates this feeling of low self-worth, of not being good enough and you kind of perpetuate that myth, I'll say by stuttering because of course, that just confirms that you are not good enough and can't do what your boss wants. So by escaping that story and starting to tell yourself a new one, it's a very valuable technique and that is one technique that I used when I couldn't meditate."

Newell would tell herself that she couldn't meditate and just like I identified myself as a stutterer she identified herself as a non-meditator. That was her experience and when she started to notice and become aware of those thoughts she would change the story in her mind and say, "I can meditate, everyone can meditate, we all are capable of meditating." She then explains, "Slowly my abilities to meditate started to turn around and so it is the stories that we tell ourselves that are so powerful and most of us aren't aware of them. So when a symptom like stuttering comes up, everyone is looking for some reason why? I would imagine that every single person with that particular issue, potentially has a slightly different reason why that it is all related to those feelings of feeling not worthy or not good enough, that is really a universal wound we all have, I would say. It comes out in different ways for each of us, in my case, rather than stuttering, I would just keep my mouth shut, I wouldn't say anything at all because I learned that if I said something and someone didn't agree with me or wanted to put me in my place, I thought "Okay, well I just save that for someone who cares" and that was the story I told myself and I would never be a public speaker, that would been the last thing I thought that I would do until I met Dr. Eben Alexander."

Newell had been avoiding speaking in public but Dr Eben Alexander insisted, "No, we are going to share this information to everyone around the world and you're going to be up there talking. Newell was steadfast in her refusal to speak in public and said, "absolutely not, I will not be up there talking with you and I don't do that."

One day, Dr Eben Alexander was invited to present a workshop and he just added Karen Newell's name to the flyer unknown to her, so suddenly she needed to speak in front of an audience. Explaining what happened next, Newell says, "when I got up to speak I didn't have any notes, I was very nervous about what I was going to say. When I got up to speak for the very first time about this topic about sound, meditation and consciousness I suddenly knew what to say. It was unbelievable how comfortable I felt in that moment. From that moment forward, I realised when I'm talking about something I'm comfortable with, when I'm talking about something I know very well through my own personal experience, something I have a lot of confidence around, I don't have any trouble at all speaking, publicly in front of audiences and that was a brand new thing for me. I'm 54 years old, I was almost 50 years old when I finally realised, "oh my gosh, I can do public speaking." So, it's never too late and we all have gifts inside and usually the things we resist most, are the things that if we can get through them, would reveal our greatest gifts."

Explaining how sound and more specifically Sacred Acoustics can help anyone to meditate, Newell says, "these sound files are very unique, they include something called brain wave entrainment, many people know them as binaural beats. Now, the tones that we create are a combination of binaural beats, monaural beats and other sound effects that we combined with the very precise harmonic principles. That's a little different than how your average binaural beat producer might create these kind of sounds. What binaural beats do is they drive signals to the brain, different frequencies that helps you bring the brain from the normal waking awareness consciousness, the beta state. That's the state we're in, where we're walking around and we are talking. The delta state, is the state that we're in when we're asleep. Theta is just up from that maybe a deep state of meditation and alpha is maybe a state of profound relaxation, profound focus, when you're really working closely on a project, flow kind of state. Now what we try to do with our tones is drive the brain down into that state between awake and asleep. That border line between delta and theta, the hypnogogic state. This state allows us to kind of let go of physical awareness of the body, of the here, of the now, the time, the space and it allows us to kind of become more aware of ourselves as pure energy, as pure vibration, the observer behind the thoughts."

Sharing the benefits of Sacred Acoustics for beginners, Newell says, "If you are a beginner, it can really help like it did for me. This kind of binaural beats technology helped to settle my racing thoughts, that beta state of awareness that is constantly thinking and then can drive to that lower state of theta. It helps the brain get calmer and so for beginners this can be quite useful."

And for advanced meditators, Newell says, "People who are already very comfortable with getting into a state of mind, where they can let go of their thinking, where they can find their quiet space inside. Many of those people tells us that our tones helped them go even deeper and they are able to, some of them, you know, visual things start to happen if they weren't happening before, connections, states that they haven't quite gotten to before, kind of gives them that little boost. Every technique is different for everyone but it's very easy to try, we offer a free 20 minute meditation on our website, SacredAcoustics.com, you go there and look for free download."

Explaining the origins of the sound 'OM' and it being the primordial sound, Newell shares, "primordial is the really the state before space and time. The place we came from, the energetic state of origin or creation. That primordial state before we were born, before we came into our bodies and the OM, as it happens, I'll tell you my personal reason for using OM. I found it in all the different classes that I took and different types of techniques that I learned. Actually vocalizing OM... or it can be any sound, really, but OM is the most common. Feeling that vibration in your throat "OMMMM" when you can feel the vibrations of your body that starts to allow you to feel the vibrational essence of who you are and this OM is a very beautiful way to bring that vibration up inside of yourself and when used in connection with the tones, it kind of allows you to create the vibration inside your body and then it kind of connects with the vibration of the tones and you can imagine your essences kind of being carried by these tones. Now many people are attached to OM for religious reasons, Hindus, OM is incredibly important to them. "

Newell adds, "Very interestingly, Eben Alexander, my co-author in Living in a Mindful Universe, during his profound near-death experience while in coma, he heard this sound OM in the deepest part of his experience, it was a deep resonance sound when he was the furthest into what he called, the core. That's the sound he heard, that was the resonance and it was so powerful to him that when he came back, he identified that energy, that presence, that deity as OM which many would call God but to him, God had too much baggage and OM for him was a very pure un-baggaged term. Now we do hear from certain people with religious beliefs who found that OM is a little threatening and what comes with that is a bunch of eastern belief systems and that, it's just not true in our case. In our case it is just a pure vibration that we make with our voice and we encourage everyone to try this for yourself and see if it does help you get even deeper in any meditative state."

Sharing how, as a person who stuttered, I was never truly aware of my stuttering experience. However now I am perfectly aware when I am speaking. Meditating has helped developed this awareness. Newell explains, "being unaware of what you're doing is pretty common in this world and its only when a problem presents itself like stuttering that we maybe want to go and figure out what's going on, so really this kinds of things I have to say are gifts. Problems that we have in our world cause us to look behind the problem and see what's going on and usually when we do that, what comes with it is an amazing spiritual growth whether that's what we meant to or not. This idea of identifying that inner observer, that inner observer can have awareness of what's going on. Multiple things can be going on at once, we are trained to kind of put our awareness on one thing, so if you're in a busy airport for example and there is a lot of announcements about flights boarding and things, you are usually still able to focus only on the person that your speaking to sitting right next to you. You can tune all that other stuff out and when we can consciously become aware of that inner observer and consciously decide what we are going to tune in to, what are we not going to tune in to. Then we can start to really get behind different problems of the day, whether its stuttering or whether it's in my case, its public speaking or whatever issues someone might have, these are our gifts. These are the things that bother us the most or the things we should be looking at, trying to uncover what's going on underneath and what comes with that is greater awareness of who we really are and really channeling that energy consciously of who we want to be."

By watching your breath and really practicing regularly how you are separate from your thoughts it is possible to develop the realization that you are the indwelling God that observes everything. Newell describes it as, "That observer within is your connection to that, I'll call it, primordial mind, what you just described is your connection and so in order to get there you must learn to quiet the mind, to find the still space inside and the beginner's stages of that are simply, watch your breath and notice how your different from your thoughts. When your thoughts starts to wander, when you're watching your breath, what is that part of you that notices, what is the part of you that watches and returns your attention to your breathing, that's the inner observer. That is your channel, your connection. Once you can get into the state in an easy fashion, it can take weeks, it may take months to get there and it very worth getting there. Once you're able to do that, that allows you to get behind that God from within that primordial mind that we are all made of, that we kind of forgotten about that we disconnected from and by consciously reconnecting to that energy, through that observer within gaining more awareness of that energetic part of you that is your path way to that primordial mind in that God force."

We are all very unique aspects of a whole and each of us have come here with different gifts and challenges. Our purpose is to rise above the challenges and bring the gifts to the forefront. The challenges are often clues to what the hidden gifts really are and Newell explains, "So this idea of loving our self, we hear this a lot, you know, very often this adage, "you can't truly love another until you love yourself" but most of us run into relationships all the time where we love the other but we really haven't been taught to love ourselves. Now loving myself was a topic that was confusing to me, 'how do direct love towards myself, if I'm myself?' And when I loved someone else I really was doing it with my mind, my thought. I had good feelings, I had good thoughts about someone and good feelings but the power of it was coming from my mind. And when I realised the power could actually come from my heart, that's what I realised what true love truly is. So this practice of feeling gratitude from within eventually led to the realisation that when I created that feeling of gratitude from within I was actually creating love from within. Gratitude and love are very similar kinds of energy."

When people talk about unconditional love, love without conditions, that's the purest form of love where it does matter what you do, who you are, stutterer, bad public speaker, whatever it is, that's all of who you are and so when we are trying to ignore part of us, Newell shares, "We are not truly accepting all of us unconditionally. That is not easy to do, so this building it from inside this allows for all of the kind of negative talk and the idea that you can build it from inside made me realise that loving myself was not really the right words to use but becoming the love that I already have within, was the way to go. So just changing the semantics for me made so much difference. When I discovered the book "be love now", that's exactly what Ram Dass was talking about and doing, he was being love so it's an action of being, becoming and not an action of doing."

On the importance of building the love from within being the ultimate golden rule, Newell says, "When we are building love within ourselves we are affecting people around us without them even realising." Commenting on how many of us really learned from someone telling us what it would be like to accomplish something Newell adds, "We need to have the experience of actually doing it before we actually know. Know, not just believe that something is real and building that love within, I guarantee you every human on the planet, this is your birth right to become that love that we were made of, the primordial mind is unconditional, its compassionate it has an understanding that "All is well", and that includes all of our challenges and hardships, all of them and that helps you understand how to become the love."

Sharing how feelings are important in the manifestation of anything in the external world, Newell says, "that the feeling state is so important, it's no surprise that it's kind of late to the party, how to bring your feelings into a manifestation because feelings have been ignored all this time as is something we want to avoid, we want to avoid all of that suffering but really those feelings are engines, beautiful engines and so I often will encourage people to come up with intentions or a sound journey or a meditation or just any moment of contemplation and that intention will be represented by just one word and so it could be a word like, success, or confidence. Whatever that is you are seeking in your life, generate a feeling of what it feels like to be confident. If you're trying to be confident in public speaking but you're not already, think of something you are already confident in like, brushing your teeth, something very simple, I'm very confident at brushing my teeth. Feel what it feels like to be confident and then with your mind you can kind of attach it to that other thing that maybe you aren't so confident at, the more you do this, the more you kind of resonate that feeling of what you want to receive, the world just resonates."

Concluding, she says, "The resonance in science like does attract like and so being that love or being that confidence or being that success in whatever that you're trying to achieve. Already believing that you're successful is absolutely going to then have the external world respond and reflect what's going on inside and really again the only way to know this is to try it yourself and it is a beautiful technique for manifesting what you want to have in your life."

I ask again, are you the voice or the awareness that is behind the voice? Make the voice say 'I love myself.' Make the voice repeat it 8 more times. Think of someone you dearly love, your mother or child for example. Remember all the great experiences you shared together. Remember the hugs. Now, close your eyes and repeat the same phrase 9 more times, but this time with emotion and feeling. Really believe you love yourself.

Thought for the Day: "'What a liberation to realise that the 'voice in my head' is not who I am. Who am I then? The one who sees that." Eckhart Tolle

Talking point: Have you examined who are you really? Are you the voice that is forever criticising everyone and everything? Or are you actually the inner being that is the observer?

DAY 92: THE RECOVERING STUTTER

For many years I thought I would always be a recovering stutterer kind of like a recovering alcoholic. And that was the way I led my life. I was a recovering stutterer but wasn't really proud of it. I don't know many people who advertise themselves as recovering alcoholics but that was the prescribed medicine on the speech therapy course. I would tell people that I was working on my speech and was a recovering stutterer, if I was having a bad speech day; and try to use all the tricks I had in my wand to stutter on purpose so I felt in control. However the horse had already bolted and I was in the stuttering jungle. It was too late. The only way out of this jungle was to re-invent myself from the bottom up and see myself living the life of my dreams despite the stutter.

I had the mindset of a recovering stutterer and thought the stutter would be my life companion. I didn't like the stutter or the part of me that stuttered. I felt ashamed of it. Despite advertising myself as a stutterer by stuttering on purpose when I was having a good speech day no real breakthrough was forthcoming. There had to be another way as I wanted to be truly free from the stuttering mind. I had the mindset of being cautious and risk averse. This was apparent in all areas of my life. I didn't have a girlfriend and was comfortable in my job. I was playing it safe.

As a recovering stutterer I would hold back in situations. Even though I could speak without stuttering that much I wouldn't speak my mind. I always had lots of things to say but the mind had somehow blocked its self from expressing. So I would always be the quiet one. This mind set would persist for another 15 years until I wrote my first book - Rich Thinking.

What changed was the realization that I hadn't truly accepted myself as a human being. I wasn't comfortable in my own skin. I wasn't happy with being a stutterer or a recovering stutterer. I still wanted to hide this secret. I was so ashamed of myself by the fact I stuttered that I didn't want people know this secret and so I led my life in such a way so as not to get noticed. However people did notice. Whenever I opened my mouth I would stutter as there was a part of my subconscious that was so scared of people noticing me it wanted to get noticed to reveal to my conscious part that I need to accept that part and be happy for the way I was. I was constantly battling to avoid getting noticed and so it was that I did get noticed.

By advertising the fact that I had a stutter and actually deciding to be open about it by stuttering on purpose, this started the process of clearing up the subconscious mind's reluctance to let go of the need to stutter.

The stutter is the inability to have control of the breath and simultaneous production of vocal sounds. It's really quite simple if you think about it. Breathe and then speak, however as a stutterer the breathing would be the first to go and the vocalization of sounds would not be possible as there would be tension in the mouth, jaw and throat regions. The combination of anxiety, lack of breathing control, vocalization of sounds and fear which led to avoidance, holding back, blocking, repetition built up over a number of years would result in a stutterer.

The stutter is a manifestation of the self-doubt I created when I started to speak. Built up over a number wasted years, this was the way I led my life, and the only reason I changed was when I started to pursue my dream irrespective of the stutter. I no longer used the stutter as an excuse. For many years, I would say to myself, 'When I stop stuttering, I will do this and that.' And truth be told - I did nothing.

Thought for the Day: "It's not what we do once in a while that shapes our lives. It's what we do consistently." Anthony Robbins.

Talking point: How long have you been a recovering stutterer? Isn't it time to make a break from the repetition of speech therapy courses and start on the inward journey?

DAY 93: FLUENT OR NON-STUTTERS

Since the day I was labelled a stutterer, it was my aim to become fluent and not to stutter. By setting such a target I had programmed myself for failure. Even Prime Minister Tony Blair, when pressed, stumbles over words. It's part of being human.

I now use the term 'non-stutterer' for the general population; people who don't have doubt in their ability to speak. That was what happened to me. Over a period of time, the self-doubt grew from an acorn into a giant stuttering tree with roots so deep that it shook the foundations of my being. It has taken me over 30 years to recover from this earthquake.

The leaves and branches show my outward appearance as being shy, nervous, quiet, stuttering, blocking, facial tics, shallow breathing, panic, and apprehension. However, when uncovering the roots, a whole new world is revealed. Doubt, depression, anger, frustration, isolation, denial, shame and worthlessness to name just a few.

The idea of not stuttering caused me to avoid pain. Being motivated not to stutter, as it was deemed to be bad, meant I was trying to unsuccessfully to avoid pain. No matter what I tried I would stutter.

I needed to examine the roots to see what was happening. I had to examine the soil, the environment, and weed out any poisonous plants. And importantly I had to water the tree with empowering beliefs.

I was a smart stutterer or so I thought. Sometimes covert or overt. Most people knew I stuttered, but occasionally, people would wonder who was the quiet one in the corner. That would be me. I would only speak when needed so felt on the outside most of my life. I was detached from the world.

I met a guy on personal development course whose name was Nifty. Like in many situations I tell people that I had a stutter and sometimes I would stumble. So, Nifty, told me he used to stutter too. But, Nifty still stuttered. Every other word that would come out of his mouth was an obvious stumble. However, he said to me, "I used to have a stutter." For me, it was interesting that in his own mind, the stutter was a non-issue. He was a successful businessman, irrespective of the stuttering behaviour and he was living his life and not letting the stutter determine his course.

Thought for the Day: "The secret of making something work in your lives is, first of all, the deep desire to make it work. Then the faith and belief that it can work. Then to hold that clear definite vision in your consciousness and see it working out step by step, without one thought of doubt or disbelief." Eileen Caddy

Talking point: If you want to be seen as a fluent speaker then the game is up. If you want to be seen as a person who is working on his speech then you are in the game. If you can be seen as a person who is living his life despite the stutter you are winning the game.

DAY 94: STUTTERING PARALYSIS

Stuttering is a result of thoughts, emotions, beliefs, perceptions and actions influenced by the environment that has been habituated over a period of time. The mis-production of sound, prefaced by the mental thought processes of what is going to be articulated, due to a block or interruption in the mental process, causes stuttering to manifest.

In the millisecond prior to speaking the subconscious searches through its database. Every single moment of our existence is stored in the subconscious mind and so the years of stuttering, the archives of fear and self-doubt will be recalled and cause the speech production process to misfire.

Consciously I did not want to stutter or have the negative experiences repeated, so the subconscious would oblige and not co-ordinate the necessary activities to enable me to speak.

As previously stressed, the brain is there to do the least amount of work and preserve the status quo. So in the case of a stutterer it was telling me to stop speaking. If you are a person who repeats sounds, syllables and words then you will be consciously trying your best to override the commands from the subconscious and failing miserably. The same applies to people who block. They are trying to force out a sound or word but the subconscious is still in charge.

I was a repeater and blocker. My subconscious was all powerful in letting me know that it was a big bad world and it was better not to speak, so when I tried to speak I would block and repeat like a parrot. However in many situations I would be the silent one, as I had learnt not to speak.

While there maybe external factors that may influence your thoughts about a situation, the truth is, you and only you are the originator of the emotional block. The block from the subconscious is sending you a message, 'stop speaking.' However consciously, you carry on, therefore the stuttering manifests. It's a constant battle between the subconscious and conscious mind that results in the stuttering. The breathing is first to go out of balance, tension in the mouth, jaw and throat areas soon follow. It's no wonder you are stuttering and will continue to do so until the subconscious is in alignment with your conscious goals.

The subconscious mind is doing what it needs to do. It's there to look after you. Remember that sabre-toothed tiger that is out lurking in the streets of London. Well, you subconscious mind is there to protect you and tell you to run, even before you see it.

Indeed 95% of your daily life is run by the subconscious. Until the age of 7, you mind was in a state of hypnosis and you copied all the programs from your parents and those who surrounded you. So if you want to change this programming you will need to repeat a new program or belief until it is installed in your subconscious.

Think of your conscious mind as the creative force. This is where your wishes and desires emanate from. The subconscious mind is a computer. It is the subconscious that creates reality. If you look around your life and see where you are having problems, you will see what subconscious beliefs are running, which in turn is creating your world around you.

In my case, as a person who stuttered, it was always be in my mind that stuttering was bad and something to be avoided. And that's the way I led my life, I would not speak, not socialise and basically not do anything. That was a conscious decision. Years of negative thought patterns in regards to stuttering changed my life for the worse.

As a person who stutters, I would 100% of the time, rehearse in my mind the situation. I wasn't an optimist, so my mind would be filled with Freddy Kruger scenes of stuttering. This pattern of thinking would remain the default irrespective of whatever I consciously tried. I needed to reprogram my subconscious mind to have lasting freedom.

Thought for the Day: "The stutterer must conquer his own problems. No one else can do it for him." Charles Van Riper

Talking point: When did you get sent to speech therapy? When did you first start to have negative emotions regarding stuttering?

DAY 95: PRICELESS

The following are three insights I gained from writing my first book that have helped me to become free.

Firstly, that separation is an illusion. You may just think that you are a human being living on this planet called Earth. However just like a drop of water is part of the ocean, you are actually part of the universe. In 1950 Albert Einstein wrote a letter to a grieving father who lost a son to Polio:

'A human being is a part of the whole, called by us "Universe," a part limited in time and space. He experiences himself, his thoughts and feelings as something separate from the rest — a kind of optical delusion of his consciousness. The striving to free oneself from this delusion is the one issue of true religion. Not to nourish it but to try to overcome it is the way to reach the attainable measure of peace of mind.'

By understanding this concept of separation as an illusion, it helped to release all the fears I had about myself and the way I speak. As a child I had no problem about stumbling over words and speaking. It was only when I was sent to speech therapy I began to think something was wrong with the way that I spoke. Having gained this insight about how we are all connected to one another and everything in the universe is Energy, how can I be judged about the way I speak? It is true that the reaction of listeners will be a challenge, and the only way I was able to become desensitised was to stutter on purpose, where I was in control of the speaking situation. It was only when I took charge and assertively spoke, that my reactions to their reactions changed, and so the healing within me started to take place. Fundamentally, I asked myself: How can I judge anyone else if they are actually a part of me? How can I fear anyone else if they are part of me? We are all part of the one universe, the one energy, the one being!

Secondly, your invisible world creates your visible world. It is with your thoughts, feelings and emotions that you create your experiences of the world. Brian Tracy says: "Your outer world is a reflection of your inner world, and it corresponds to your dominant patterns of thinking. You become what you think about most of the time. Change your thinking, and you will change your life."

For a long time, I used to enter into speaking situations with the voice in my head wondering if I would stutter. I would build the situation so big in my head, that I would become paralysed and would avoid it. I avoided doing presentations by missing class. I avoided asking girls out and avoided rejection. I was Mr Avoid and life was passing me by.

Just by having this mind virus where I would doubt my ability to speak, the stutter manifested. Even though I had been on the speech therapy programme for many years I would still have that thought. My breakthrough came at the point when I went travelling. I learnt Spanish and went to South America. While travelling I met a lot of new people and for the first time in my life, I enjoyed talking. Even though I stuttered here and there, it did not bother me. I was no longer the shy 15 year old who wouldn't say a word for fear of stuttering out loud. I was no longer holding back. I was saying Yes to life!

I could always read out loud or speak out loud when by myself. The stutter would come out when I was in the company of others. So I concluded there was nothing wrong with my speaking process that could not be dealt with by addressing the incorrect breathing, stress and anxiety which manifested itself as stuttering when I was with other people. I know now it was just the thought of stuttering which created the fear of stuttering, and what actually happened was that I stuttered. There is nothing to fear other than fear itself.

Thirdly, be happy and grateful for what you have. Look around you, there are countless others who are worse off than you are. Be really thankful for the life that you lead. If you can be really happy and grateful then the reality creation process will be easier. I believe that if you can see the truth that everything in the world is made up of energy, then by being happy, the universe will have your back and experience life through you.

Thought for the Day: "I believe that we are solely responsible for our choices, and we have to accept the consequences of every deed, word, and thought throughout our lifetime." Elizabeth Kubler-Ross

Talking point: If you can truly embrace the three insights in this chapter you will be on the way to freedom. Meditate on them. Contemplate to them. Make them part of your life and you will see results.

DAY 96: THE POWER WITHIN

The mind is the greatest instrument the creator gave you. With the power of your mind you can create your reality. In my first book, Rich Thinking, Richard Schultz, explains how the conscious mind is fundamentally responsible for reasoning; it's that part of you which makes decisions out of choices. And it is open to having new experiences. For example you consciously decide to learn a new language or take up belly dancing. The conscious mind, known as the gatekeeper, guards the doorway to the subconscious mind. At the time of the earliest evolution of man, it is as if we had been programmed and were simply running on automatic pilot for everything. In the past we would rely on the subconscious. Rather than making conscious choices, the subconscious used to define everything that we did.

Schultz continues "Now, however, we are in the age of consciousness. We are designed to make choices: we choose our direction and our goals. We have the ability to play with decisions and choices and that is where the real power is.

The conscious mind makes the decision, and, based on this, everything will change. We are consciously choosing to be aware, to be awake."

This is supported by inventor, Nikola Tesla, who said: "My brain is only a receiver; in the universe there is a core from which we obtain knowledge, strength and inspiration. I have not penetrated into the secrets of this core, but I know that it exists."

On the other hand the subconscious mind likes familiar things; 95% of your daily life is run by the subconscious mind on autopilot. It manages your breathing and blood flow and keeps you safe. If you are going to transform your life, you need to remove the limiting beliefs to reach your goals, and you need to make these changes at the subconscious level.

When you are walking into a new situation, your subconscious mind will assess if it's safe to stay there. Sometimes you may feel stressed in a particular environment without knowing why. It could be that your subconscious mind is processing events in the background before you are consciously aware of them. It is said that the subconscious mind is a million times more powerful than the conscious mind.

If you have a goal and the subconscious mind doesn't think it is feasible, the conscious mind has no chance of achieving it. That's why sometimes you procrastinate, sabotage yourself and you're not able to move forward at all. It's normal behaviour, but it can be addressed. This is due to having limiting beliefs at the level of the subconscious mind, which holds you, or in a worst case scenario, pushes you in the opposite direction.

If you get the subconscious mind to work in partnership with the conscious mind, then almost anything is attainable. It is highly important that you have the subconscious mind on board with the goals of the conscious mind if you are going to achieve your life's dreams.

The subconscious mind is like a small child – you need to tell it exactly what it wants and explain how things should look, sound, feel, smell and taste. You need to literally describe the full experience and you will be there in that moment.

The subconscious mind is in an eternal timeless present time state where everything is happening right now. For example, if there is someone who owes you money, you can feel the stress right now, and the tension increases even as you think about that person. It's as if it's happening right now. You are in that very moment experiencing that emotion, and it fills your whole body with anger and stress.

The conscious mind, on the other hand, is time-bound, either in the past or the future, where you review memories and think about what happened last week, or you are day-dreaming as to how the next interaction with that person will go.

The stutter must therefore be at the subconscious mind level which is why I used to get so nervous and anxious whenever entering into a situation I perceived as dangerous. Consciously I am aware that speaking to someone does not threaten my life, but my breathing and anxiety levels say otherwise and these are both controlled by the subconscious.

Our reality, then, is created primarily from the subconscious, which does this on automatic and on a consistent basis. Our subconscious likes habit and consistency. Our real power, however, is found in our conscious mind.

By using breathing techniques and voice production methods this is one way to be conscious when speaking. Schultz expands:

"To make changes to the subconscious requires a ritual and for some it make need to be longer in duration and more intense. This would depend on the strength of the mind. For example they might need to repeat an affirmation every day for three months however in some cases this can be much quicker. If on the other hand, belief systems about how easy it is to develop the connection with the subconscious mind, may allow changes to be made instantly."

Meditation and strategies of being in the right state of mind, and making use of Alpha, Theta and Delta brain waves can also be useful in reprogramming the subconscious mind. The brainwave states put you in an optimum feeling of relaxation, where learning and higher thinking can take place.

The reprogramming of the subconscious mind can happen really quickly if you can make a decision. However affirmations tend to be slower.

Being happy with your current reality, makes the process of reality creation easier, and success faster. However most of us have got into the habit of doing things, in order to have things, in order to achieve happiness. This is a mechanism of cause and effect: if we do things, we will get things or experiences, and then we will be happy. What we are doing, then, is delaying our happiness until we reach the end of this process; and what often happens is that we get caught up in the doing stage.

Schultz continues, "This method of reality creation can work fairly well in a world where you have managed to achieve your goals – you feel a sense of success because you have reached your goal – but it would be better still if you can, in your conscious mind, make the decision to feel happy, regardless."

Schultz concludes, "All of us have had experiences of feeling successful or happy whether it was something small or something huge. If you can take that memory of being happy and feel it in the body as much as possible, build it up, sing and dance to it and really get into that felling then reality creation will be easy. Then you will find inspiration flow from you. Instead of feeling pessimistic you will be inspired to carry on."

Thought for the Day: "Passion is energy. Feel the power that comes from focusing on what excites you." Oprah Winfrey.

Talking point: There is immense power within each and every one of us. It is for us to believe and cultivate this feeling. Whatever you truly believe can and will be manifested.

DAY 97: HOLOGRAM

In the prequel book for The Stuttering Mind Series, Rich Thinking - 66 Days To Freedom, New York Times bestselling author Mark Anastasi, shares "The world's most advanced scientists and quantum physicists have come to the conclusion that physical matter is an illusion. There is no such thing as physical matter in our universe – there is only energy. When they looked at the smallest atoms that constitute what we think of as matter; and took the nucleus of the atoms, and opened up the neutrons inside them and the electrons that constantly zip in and out of reality around the nucleus. They wanted to find out what in that matter is physically solid and real. What they found, however, was nothing – there is no such thing as solid, physical reality. Everything is just an illusion caused by our senses. We think of our universe as being physical and real, but in actual fact it contains nothing physical at all."

"How can you explain this massive contradiction at the heart of science?" asks Anastasi. "Scientists have said that all matter is but empty space with a pattern of energy running through it. A singular pattern of energy." Everything, from the furthest star in our galaxy and every other star, every galaxy and every planet, to our planet and everything on it, every person, every object and item of furniture in your house, and even the very air that we breathe – is all nothing but one big energy field.

The only thing that scientists can compare it to, Anastasi says, is a thought wave – which begs the question: whose thought wave is it? An interesting point to ponder.

Ever since the dawn of time, mystics have been saying that we are all part of the mind of God. There is a creator, Anastasi explains, a supreme intelligence, and the mind of this supreme intellect started vibrating, generating thought energy. Faster and faster it vibrated, making the thought energy become denser and denser, more and more compacted and amalgamated, until that thought energy became what we know as physical matter. It exploded it into physical reality, in what scientists have called the Big Bang.

If we accept that matter is an illusion – whether this is because of the evidence of science and quantum physics or because of the theories of metaphysics and an understanding of the spirit world – then we will also understand that the concept of separation between human beings is also an illusion. Everyone, Ansatasi says, "is a part of the same body; we are all part of the same mind, which is manifesting itself through this reality that we see as physical."

He continues, "It's figuring out what it is through us, through our self-expressions, through our choices." This also means, that we can never really die. If we are energy, then we are immortal – an eternal energy that will just keep on manifesting itself and being created anew, just in a different physical manifestation each time.

"You die, you go back to where you come from and then afterwards you choose to come back to physical reality to learn something new, to experience something new, to learn how to love more," says Anastasi.

In 2005, when he realised this, Anastasi says that he was able to understand that there is no separation. If he was to walk into a bookstore or a supermarket, for example, or host a seminar, he would see that all the people in the bookstore or supermarket, all the people in the seminar, "are me."

This realisation increased his confidence. "If I'm in front of 500 people," he says, "and they are me and I'm them, how can there be judgement? There can't be judgement because I would just be judging myself, which is ridiculous – they would just be judging themselves. It's just one part of me speaking to other parts of me, healing other parts of me."

Another aspect of this is the idea that everyone present had agreed before coming that they would meet on that particular day; they had agreed on what role everyone would play. It had all been agreed that they would share the experience together, and that they would go on and move forward together.

This experience of Anastasi's made him think of an experience he remembered from when he was about six years old and he was playing with Lego. It was a childhood memory which seemed to connect with what he was experiencing as a young man in his 20s; ultimately it helped him to blossom in his business. It seemed to him to be an allegory, a story about the creation of the universe.

By its very nature, Lego involves creating and destroying, then creating and destroying again, and to Anastasi as a child, just following the instructions to build the lunar space station and then destroying it again became boring to him. As he played, he made up stories, creating little scenarios in his head. He was playing with five Lego men, making them attack and take over a lunar space station. In enacting this story as he played, he was putting a little part of his consciousness into the Lego men to enable them to act out the scenario.

At the seminar in 2005, as he listened to the talk, he remembered doing this with the Lego, and it just seemed to make sense to him. As a 6-year-old child, he had been the creator of that lunar surface, the Lego figures' playground, and, as he had grown bored of just creating, he had enabled those Lego men to 'live' through a part of his consciousness. If the little Lego men had been able to do so, they might have thought themselves to be alive, and they might have pictured themselves as individuals, thought that they were separate, when in reality they were all just a part of their creator's consciousness.

At the talk in 2005, then, the speaker had said that there was a consciousness that created, destroyed and then re-created a playground. Because nothing happened in that playground, the consciousness found it boring because nothing was at stake. If someone is in a situation where they think that they might die, then this is when something is at stake, and this is when it is possible to really live – to experience life as a whole rainbow spectrum of emotions that keeps you at the edge of your seat.

Death itself is an illusion – we are eternal, immortal, we are all part of one another, so in reality we can never die. However, if, in our physical reality, we are facing the illusion of death, then this is when we will really experience life at its fullest – both the ups the downs, both the good and the bad, both the light and the dark, the pain and everything else that is connected to this life.

From that moment onward, for Anastasi, things all made sense. He felt confident to do seminars in front of large groups of people, because he felt that he was connected with everyone else in the room. "I didn't fear what they think of me, or what anybody thinks of me," he says, "because there isn't anybody else outside me – there's just me, and everyone is part of me and I'm part of everyone else. It's just me."

This is his message to everyone: "It's just you, and you're playing out a game. You're eternal; you're never going to die." Physical reality, he stresses, is all no more than an illusion.

Similarly when I realised that we are all part of the one being and in fact all the human beings are also part of the same 'One' being, the fear of stuttering and fear of being judged went away. This insight from Mark Anastasi had a profound impact on the way I looked at the world.

Relating this to stuttering, I could see the beliefs I had about reality were no longer correct. Just like our ancestors once thought that the sun revolved around the Earth and later discovered it was incorrect; I had discovered that the stuttering mindset of separation and doubt to be incorrect.

Thought for the Day: "If you propose to speak, always ask yourself - is it true, is it necessary, is it kind?" Buddha

Talking point: Are you able to imagine the possibility of living in the Matrix where you can literally create the life of your dreams?

DAY 98: MANIFESTING REALITY

I used to day dream all the time, aimlessly. My teenage years were a waste of time. I would recount experiences and fantasize about my life. However, now I visualize. What is the difference, you ask? Well, it is the focused concentration of an ideal outcome already present in life. Believing in the desired outcome, almost to the point of obsession that it will come to pass, is critical to the manifestation. And then, letting go of the need to have it come to fruition. The key is to be happy irrespective of whether it comes to pass.

Each night we die, when we enter sleep we pass from our conscious state into the subconscious. This is akin to death. It's like we are transported to another dimension. A place, where all things exist, and time has no meaning. You dream of loved ones and adventures in far off places. And, we hopefully wake up the following morning. What happens during the eight or so hours of sleep? In a 24 hour period, we spend a third of that sleeping. Could this provide us with a clue as to the reality of life? What if we could use dreams to create what happens during our sleep state to manifest into the other 16 hour period where we are supposedly awake?

In this dream state, the subconscious is active. It is processing all the data since its previous download. All your day's activities and experiences are being evaluated and processed. Occasionally, you may recall dreams the following morning. What if it's possible to interrupt this programming and consciously choose what the subconscious does during those eight hours? Could you with your thoughts, emotions and feelings interject into the subconscious mind your deepest wishes and desires? I believe so. I have been using subliminal audio messages for a while, just before going to sleep, to reprogram my mind. It is said, as one enters sleep, the brain is at its most receptive to suggestion.

If you are agitated, irritated or cannot settle down to a good night's sleep, it would be best to get up out of bed and do something to take your mind off it. This could be reading an inspirational book such as Rich Thinking, or listening to some relaxing music or even remembering the things you are most grateful for. What you do just before you sleep is probably the most important thing you can do if you want to live an inspired life.

As a person who stuttered, I said affirmations such as I am a powerful, eloquent and confident speaker. I am at ease speaking in front of people. I am in perfect control of my speech. I am having fun speaking. I am enjoying talking to new people.

The subconscious mind cannot tell the difference between what is real and what was imagined. You can choose to review the events and drama of the day or choose to sow seeds of growth and empowerment. It doesn't really matter to your subconscious. It is like a computer, waiting for your programming instructions and so each night before you go to sleep you have a choice.

So if you had a bad speech day, then imagine or remember a day that you were in perfect control of your speech. It could be when you gave a speech at your sister's wedding. You remember you spoke with such eloquence and confidence and the guests even laughed at your jokes. You see yourself having a fun time speaking. Really remember the moment. Feel the feelings of confidence you had when speaking that day. Hear the power of your voice and smell the room where you are at. Really savour the wedding cake. Touch your heart and be immensely grateful for the experience of delivering a speech at your sister's wedding.

By using all six senses including that of feeling the feelings of speaking with control, when you are about to sleep you will be able to program your subconscious into this way of being. Assume you have your deepest wish of speaking with eloquence and confidence as you dose off to sleep, already realised and you will dream it into existence.

My first clue to a life without stuttering came in 2008, when I had a telephone interview for a job in Bermuda. I aced it, and they offered me the job while on the call. I had my good friend, Simon, listening in to the conversation. I found out quite early on, that whenever I had someone who stuttered, listening in to a phone call, the speech production would be effortless and without stress. That led me to believe that the stuttering is an inside job. For reasons, only known to my subconscious, I had developed doubt in my ability to speak, and the external environment reinforced those thoughts, so consequently I stuttered. This mindset of stuttering would be with me for over 30 years. Why? Well, I never actually took the time to re-evaluate my beliefs. It was my firm belief I would remain a recovering stutterer. Even, today it amazes me how much I enjoy speaking with complete strangers. And smiling too, I get smiles back all the time. It helps having a 2-year old son, who is a bundle of joy walking, and this reminds me that life is wonderful and should be explored, and not one that is full of self-doubt and fear.

Thought for the Day: "You are what you are by what you believe." Oprah Winfrey

Talking point: Do you really believe you can really change your way of speaking?

DAY 99: MATRIX RELOADED

s life a nightmare or a dream or neither? What if we woke up from this state to realise the truth? Could shinning a flashlight on the Matrix open up the reality of life?

Anita Moorjani, shares in her book, "Dying To Be Me," her story of how she was given 36 hours to live after being diagnosed with Cancer. She tells of her near death experience and seeing that nothing is solid and everything is Energy. In this state she experienced a complete feeling of unconditional love, saw why she got the cancer and what her role was to be in this lifetime.

In her own words, Moorjani explains, "They started me on a chemotherapy drip as well as oxygen, and then they started to take tests, particularly on my organ functions, so that they could determine what drugs to use. I was drifting in and out of consciousness during this time, and I could feel my spirit actually leaving my body. Then I actually 'crossed over' to another dimension, where I was engulfed in a total feeling of love. I also experienced extreme clarity of why I had the cancer, why I had come into this life in the first place, what role everyone in my family played in my life in the grand scheme of things, and generally how life works. The clarity and understanding I obtained in this state is almost indescribable. Words seem to limit the experience - I was at a place where I understood how much more there is than what we are able to conceive in our three-dimensional world. I realised what a gift life was, and that I was surrounded by loving spiritual beings, who were always around me even when I did not know it. The amount of love I felt was overwhelming, and from this perspective, I knew how powerful I am, and saw the amazing possibilities we as humans are capable of achieving during a physical life."

Moorjani adds, "I found out that my purpose now would be to live 'Heaven on Earth' using this new understanding, and to share this knowledge with other people. However, I had the choice of whether to come back into life, or go towards death. I was made to understand that it was not my time, but I always had the choice, and if I chose death, I would not be experiencing a lot of the gifts that the rest of my life still held in store. One of the things I wanted to know was that if I chose life, would I have to come back to this sick body, because my body was very, very sick and the organs had stopped functioning. I was then made to understand that if I chose life, my body would heal very quickly. I would see a difference in not months or weeks, but days! I was shown how illnesses start on an energetic level before they become physical. If I chose to go into life, the cancer would be gone from my energy, and my physical body would catch up very quickly. I then understood that when people have medical treatments for illnesses, it rids the illness only from their body but not from their energy so the illness returns."

Continuing Moorjani, shares "I realised if I went back, it would be with a very healthy energy. Then the physical body would catch up to the energetic conditions very quickly and permanently. I was given the understanding that this applies to anything, not only illnesses - physical conditions, psychological conditions, etc. I was 'shown' that everything going on in our lives was dependent on this energy around us, created by us. Nothing was solid - we created our surroundings, our conditions, etc. depending where this 'energy' was at.

Moorjani, excitedly explaining further says, "The clarity I received around how we get what we do was phenomenal! It's all about where we are energetically. I was made to feel that I was going to see 'proof' of this first hand if I returned back to my body. I know I was drifting in and out between the two worlds, but every time I drifted into the 'other side', I was shown more and more scenes. There was one, which showed how my life had touched all the people in it - it was sort of like a tapestry and showed how I affected everyone's lives around me. I was made to understand that, as tests had been taken for my organ functions (and the results were not out yet), that if I chose life, the results would show that my organs were functioning normally. If I chose death, the results would show organ failure as the cause of death, due to cancer."

Moorjani explains, "I was able to change the outcome of the tests by my choice! I made my choice. The doctors were unable to understand what was going on, they made me undergo test after test. I had a full body scan, and because they could not find anything, they made the radiologist repeat it again!"

Concluding Moorjani says, "Because of my experience, I am now sharing with everyone I know that miracles are possible in your life every day. After what I have seen, I realise that absolutely anything is possible, and that we did not come here to suffer. Life is supposed to be great, and we are very, very loved. The way I look at life has changed dramatically, and I am so glad to have been given a second chance to experience 'Heaven on Earth.'"

On the subject of Time as an illusion and where all things exist, Moorjani explains, "Time seems to have a completely different meaning on that side. What I felt was that all possibilities exist simultaneously - it just depends which one you choose. Sort of like being in an elevator, where all the floors of a building exist, but you can choose which floor to get off on. So if all the future possibilities exist for me to choose from, then I assume all the past scenarios exist too. So depending which future possibility I choose, that will also determine which past automatically comes with it (I chose life, so it affected the past, choosing the appropriate test result for the organ function)."

Moorjani carries on saying, "When I was being presented the choice, I actually saw a vision of my lab report, which said, on the heading: Diagnosis: Organ Failure. Then on the body of the report: Death due to organ failure caused by Hodgkin's lymphoma. When I actually saw the report after coming back, the sheet of paper looked almost identical, and the heading matched word for word: Diagnosis: Organ Failure, however, the body read: There is no evidence of organ failure. I actually got goose bumps looking at that report, knowing what it could have read."

Explaining that now Moorjani feels that everything is not real and it makes her feel very powerful, she says, "I now know that a lot more exists than we are consciously aware of or capable of understanding. Imagine there is a huge warehouse, which is dark, and you live in this warehouse with one flashlight. Everything you know about this warehouse is seen through the light of this one small flashlight. Whenever you want to look for something, you may or may not find it, but it does not mean the thing does not exist. It is there, but you just haven't flashed your light on it. You can only see what your light is focused on. Then one day, someone flicks on a light switch, and for the first time, you can see the whole warehouse. The vastness of it is almost overwhelming, you can't see all the way to the end, and you know there is more than what you can see. But you do see how all the products are lined up on all the shelves, and you notice just how many different things there are in the warehouse which you never noticed, never even conceived having existed, yet they do, simultaneously with the things you know existed (those are the things your flashlight had been able to find). Then, even when the light switch goes back off, nothing can take away the understanding and clarity of your experience. Even though you are back to one flashlight, you now know how to look for things. You know what is possible, and you even know what to look for. You start viewing things differently, and it is from this new springboard that your experiences start to happen. And so I find that in my daily life, I am referring to different aspects of my experience at different times, and I am understanding things in a different way, and knowing things I did not know I knew."

Moorjani explains, "I saw all people as 'energy', and depending where our energy level was, that was the world we created for ourselves. The understanding I gained from this was that if cancer was not in our 'energy', then it was not in our reality. If feeling good about ourselves was in our energy, then our reality would be positive. If cancer was in our energy, then even if we eradicated it with modern medicine, it would soon come back. But if we cleared it from our energy, the physical body would soon follow. None of us are as 'real' or physical as we think we are. From what I saw, it looked like we are energy first, and physical is only a result of expressing our energy. And we can change our physical reality if we change our energy. I was made to feel that in order to keep my energy/vibration level up, I only had to live in the moment, enjoy every moment of life, and use each moment to elevate the next moment (which then elevates my future). It is in that moment of elevating your energy level that you can change your future (like my test results)."

In the famous 'Double Split' experiment it was shown that an electron can be both a particle and wave; however what got physicists baffled was when the electron was being observed it behaved differently to how it acted when nothing was observing it. It was like the electron was aware of something looking at it and behaved in a certain way; but when it was aware nothing was observing it the electron acted like how it was supposed to. And even more strangely when the observer had a thought of observing it but didn't actually observe the experiment the election behaved as if it was being observed. It was like the thought affected how the election behaved. How is this possible? Welcome to the wonderful world of quantum physics where the smallest things in the universe meets consciousness.

Does this mean our thoughts create reality? This will be focus in Book 3, Realising Stuttering Freedom, of The Stuttering Mind series. If indeed life isn't what it appears to be and everything is energy, the pain of stuttering isn't what is appears to be. The stuttering made me question the reality of this world. Why could I read out perfectly well alone and yet in front of others I would stutter uncontrollably?

Thought for the Day: "Be the change you want to see in the world." Mahatma Gandhi

Talking point: If indeed we are nothing but Energy, then why are we trapped in the illusion of separation and as a result have suffered from stuttering. Realising that the whole world is nothing but an illusion created by the brain, then stuttering freedom is literally a dream away. Are you able to dream the possibility of living a life free from stuttering? Once you are able to dream stuttering freedom then you will be able to experience stuttering freedom.

EPILOGUE

As a person who stuttered, I had zero confidence, no self-esteem and countless limiting beliefs. I felt I had nothing to share with world. I felt unworthy of love. And indeed that was my reality. I didn't have a girlfriend until my thirties. I was lost in my own world of self-loathing, fear and loneliness.

The years of regret due to having a stutter brings tears to my eyes. I was a caught up in my own drama of fear, self-doubt and suicidal thoughts to do anything about it. The biggest regret was not taking a road. That road could have led me to freedom much earlier. However I was too scared. Ten years on, I decided to take that road, but alas I found that the first secret love of my life had died in a car accident three years previously. I use the word "secret", as I never told her how I felt. I just couldn't see how anyone could be interested in me. After all, I had a stutter and couldn't talk properly. So why would anyone want to go out with me. This thinking was imprinted on my psyche for a very, very long time.

In a world where the power of speech is a necessity, just like food and water, the lack of which will makes one's life intolerable. It is my mission to lift the illusion of separation, so as to share with the world that we are not separate human beings, but instead we are part of the Divine. Each and every one of us has a role to play in this drama called life, to help transform one another to be the best version we can be.

If I had realised this as a child, then the years of loneliness would have been replaced with years of friendship and love. As children, we think the world revolves around us. We felt the pain of separation, the first day we went to school, away from our mothers and fathers. This pain felt so real. We feel we are alone, but the truth of it is we are never alone. We never actually separated from the creator. It was just a cruel illusion to make the pain deeper and the sense of separation profound.

I no longer feel the need to stutter on a day to day basis. Writing this book has confirmed the transformation that has taken place. I feel truly connected to the universe and everyone in it. I am no longer afraid. How can I be afraid of myself? I can feel we are all connected through an invisible spirit. What we see with our eyes is limited. There is a whole world of Energy around us.

Whenever I have a stumble, I now class it as a stumble and nothing more. As a person who stuttered, I had often felt it necessary to over analyse any lapses in speech production. I would spend hours, days and even weeks replaying a bad speech moment over and over in my head. This is no longer the case.

Life is inherently meaningless. It is you that gives meaning to events. Things are always happening. Be it if someone didn't say, 'Good Morning' to you and your mind starts on overdrive. I recall the story of three children being rowdy playing on a bus, and the dad was just watching them. Some of the other passengers started to get irritated by the commotion and asked to dad to get the children to be quiet. When the dad explained that their mother had just died, the passengers felt sorry and bad for complaining. It is interesting to note that in a population of 7 billion people that there will always be events that occur and it is how you interpret them which will mirror your reality.

How can you be afraid of the world when there is really only you? If you are lucky to be a father or mother, then look at your son or daughter. Close your eyes and feel them next to you as you hold them close. Watch the movements in their body as they fall sleep. Do you realise that you are breathing the very same air as them? Do you ever imagine looking at the world through their eyes? Is it possible that there is only *one being* that is looking through the eyes of seven billion people and experiencing itself through the eyes? Imagine if this being gave you the power to create the life of your dreams. Just suppose, this being did, but you forgot that you had this superpower. Is it possible that you have been looking at this life through a lens of a child that has got an outdated model? It was only a few hundred years ago that people thought the Earth was flat and if a ship sailed far enough it would fall off. Similarly, it was thought that the Sun revolved around the Earth. Imagine if the creator gave you this power, all you had to do was to dream it, become aware of it, realise it and experience it. Then you will have learnt the secret to life.

This is an old Indian story that Don Miguel Ruiz recounted in his book, The Mastery of Love, in which he shares how Brahma, the name of the Supreme one energy, God was lonely so he created a beautiful goddess of illusion, Maya for the purpose of having fun. Brahma told Maya why he created her to which she replied, "Let's play a wonderful game but you will have to do as I say." Brahma agreed and created the whole universe, the sun, stars, moons and planets. Then, life on Earth: the animals, the oceans, the atmosphere, everything. Maya then remarked, "How beautiful is this world of illusion you created, now I want you to create a kind of animal that is so intelligent and aware that is can appreciate your creation". Finally, Brahma created humans. Once he finished with the creation, he asked Maya when the game was going to begin. "We'll start it immediately," she said.

Maya cut Brahma into thousands of bits and placed a little piece of Brahma in each human being and said, "Now the game begins! I am going to make you forget what you are, and you are going to try to find yourself!" Maya created the dream and that is why the universe exists. Brahma in the game of life is still trying to remember who he is.

Brahma is inside of each and every one of us. We are all part of the divine, but Maya is preventing you from remembering who are really are.

As a stutterer, my model of reality was one that meant the world was something to be feared. It was a model that I created as a child that supposedly served me. However, as a 42 year old, this model is now outdated and needs to be upgraded. Just like an old iPhone has been slowed down by the clever people at Macworld, and you need to get a brand new iPhone X as a result, the stuttering habit no longer served me and so I have upgraded my model of the world. This model is one that is loving, kind, supportive where I love meeting and talking to people. Think of the person who is a glass half full kind of person. This person will always look at the world with an optimistic perspective. In contrast, a half empty glass person, his world will be pessimistic and that will be his reality through life. It is with your beliefs that you create your world. By transforming your beliefs your life will be unimaginably beautiful.

Imagine the possibility, there is a *you* that is already free from the stuttering mind. If indeed as Einstein said, "People like us, who believe in physics, know that the distinction between past, present, and future is only a stubbornly persistent illusion." And "The only reason for time is so that everything doesn't happen at once."

Does this mean all things and events actually exist concurrently, and you can actually choose to draw towards you the experience you want to bring forth in this reality?

There is only the now, meaning you have already freed yourself from the stuttering mindset and with your beliefs you can bring it forth into this reality. I had a dream that I would speak in front of thousands of people. I had a dream that I would inspire millions. I know that everything is possible in Divine time.

In book two, of the 'The Stuttering Mind' series we will explore how your thoughts, beliefs, feelings, perceptions, emotions, habits and actions have created your reality of stuttering.

In book three, we delve into the metaphysical world of reality and relate how when you become aware of the infinite possibilities of life you no longer need to stutter or limit yourself. You are in fact perfection itself.

In book four, we will tie it all together so you can experience stuttering freedom. If you can speak in one situation, you can speak in all situations. Stuttering is an inside job.

What is your motivation for not stuttering? If it is to be seen as a 'normal' person and a fluent speaker, then it is a very slippery slope indeed. For 16 long and wasted years I was a on a speech therapy program for recovering stutterers and I would still be on it, if I hadn't got out of the mentality of wanting to work on my speech. I would religiously costal breathe for 20 minutes a day, only to find when I entered into any pressurized situation, the speaking process would fail. I was obsessed with wanting to be in control of my speech, but only when I started to live life, the speech improved as a by-product.

I haven't done any 20 minute breathing exercises for more than 10 years and there is no reason for me to return to being obsessed with working on my speech. I call it the fluency pit hole. Within the first year of the programme, I had gained all what I truly needed. The co-dependency that resulted in years of repeat courses meant I was addicted to going back for a fix. The highs of artificially being able to speak and then later on, the lows of being an out of control stutterer meant I wasn't living. I was disillusioned, disempowered and disappointed with the programme and myself for not being able to speak with freedom in real life situations.

I was not congruent with myself. One part, wanted to appear as someone who was confident and able to speak, but in the depths of my heart I wasn't happy to be a part of this world. I hadn't realised or felt connected to the universe. I felt the pain of separation to be so real and that was the way I lived my life.

As a person who stuttered, the image I had about myself was one that wasn't empowering. My way of being was based on this self-image. The idea of changing the self-image is one that can be traumatic, for the ego believes, it is the source of creation. Dr Wayne Dyer defined ego as edged God out, and so the ego will do whatever is necessary to maintain its illusion that it's correct.

The very idea of the world being different to how you think it is, will threaten the very existence of your ego. Whenever you get your button pushed, your emotions are being brought to the surface. These are subconscious memories that have been locked deep inside, it's stirring and resultant upheaval causes transformation. If an idea, deemed to be so fundamentally different that will cause a paradigm shift in your being, this is what will give you freedom.

If you are a stutterer you need to examine your beliefs such that you are able to break free from whatever excuse that your Ego comes up with. I am sure that there will be many like there were for me. It's the natural way of being. Remember you are on autopilot for 95% of the time. The subconscious likes routine so to break the habit of stuttering, you will need to revaluate what you have believed to be true.

If you are not committed to do whatever it takes to rid this way of speaking then it will be your companion forever. To be perfectly honest, I wasn't committed to doing whatever it took to transform my inner game. I was content with my life. There was nothing scary, that pushed me out of my comfort zone, and so I remained a recovering stutterer for a long time, always working on my speech. I am happy to say this is no longer the case. I am living life.

As I complete this book, a thought entered my consciousness. Would not having a stutter have meant I would not have sat on the sidelines of life? Was it the sitting on the sidelines that created the stutter?

AWARENESS

The following is an extract from Book 2, Awareness of Stuttering Freedom part of The Stuttering Mind book series due to be published in Spring 2019.

To be conscious is to be aware. The question is to be aware of what? We can only see a very small part of what is actually going on, so that means there is far more than meets the eye. What we see may not actually be the whole truth and nothing but the truth. It is our version of the truth.

My reality of stuttering was based entirely on my thoughts, emotions, feelings, perceptions, beliefs, habits, environment and actions. This stuttering pyramid, constructed and built within my own mind, created the stuttering that existed for over 30 years. When this was deconstructed the stuttering dissipated and now I don't feel the need to stutter. That part of me, which wanted to hide behind the stutter, has become free to express itself. It is on the journey inside that freedom beckons. Getting rid of the stutter without treating the underlying issues will only make the stutter resurface. That was my story based on many years in speech therapy.

Our reality is created primarily from the subconscious, which does this on automatic and on a consistent basis. Our subconscious likes habit and consistency. Our real power, therefore, is found in our conscious mind, because by choosing to have a conscious relationship with the subconscious mind we can re-programme it so that it's does different things on automatic. My new way of expressing itself free from self-doubt and fear, has now become automatic.

Becoming aware of these automatic processes is the first step to freedom. As previously established, 95 percent of our lives run on automatic. This includes speaking or stuttering as in my case. The habituated way I spoke due to self-doubt and fear meant I stuttered on automatic. It wasn't a conscious decision. When I opened my mouth to speak I stuttered. This was how it was. Try as I might, to consciously control the process proved mentally and physically exhausting. I would attend speech therapy courses and come back absolutely shattered. And, then a few days later the speech would return to its normal habituated pattern of stuttering. This course of events would be repeated over a number of years. I hadn't started working on the underlying issues of self-esteem, self-love, lack of confidence, belief and worthiness. When I did, miracles took place. The stuttering mind stopped stuttering before the stutter stopped. It was a gradual process over a number of years that resulted in interviewing 20 people to write my first book. It was only during the writing and editing that I had assimilated the insights and released all the subconscious fears that were holding me back. Upon reviewing the interviews it was apparent that I no longer stuttered, much to my surprise, and when I noticed a blip in the speech I classed it as a stumble, nothing more!

I always had a thought of, "Why is that I can speak when I am alone, and yet when in front of people, I couldn't?" That thought would resonate around my head for a few years. I hadn't found the answer, until now!

It was my belief. I had a belief that I could read and speak perfectly well when I was alone. I don't know where it came from. But what mattered was I believed it to be true. And, so that was the case. I have come across a few stutterers, who can't read aloud or speak aloud when on their own. So in their reality, the stutter is all pervasive, without exceptions.

After going on a 3-day intensive speech therapy course in 2001, I realised quite soon I could speak perfectly well to other stutterers. I had no fear. And yet other stutterers, on that and other programs, struggled with their speech with everyone. I had never thought about that previously. I wasn't aware of how my speech was, in different situations. I just knew I was a stutterer - all the time. However, looking back, I was able to speak without stuttering too much with my mother.

In recent years I could make presentations in front of people without any major worry or drama. I had developed a belief of, "When I am the centre of attention, I can speak." Public speaking is the number one fear of adults. As a person who stuttered I did not have that fear anymore. But, put me in front of a small group of 2 or 3 people I would be the proverbial wallflower.

A friend relayed a story to me of how someone he knew who was working on their speech was organising a business meeting. At the event, his boss told him to bring on his 'A game.' This had a profound impact on that person who ended up stuttering out of control for the entire session. A seemingly insignificant comment resulted in this person being ambushed and held up at gunpoint by the stutter. Previously, his speech was in control as he was comfortable speaking. And yet, two words from his boss knocked out the belief he had been developing about himself, and he was back to day zero. His environment wasn't supportive, so he stuttered uncontrollably. He had regressed back to his childhood and handed all the power to the world, and retained none.

Similarly, when working at the Prime Minister's Office, I felt I needed to impress. Although I spoke with control, the majority of my time was spent being self-conscious. I wasn't comfortable in my own skin. I wasn't confident in myself.

My self-esteem was rock bottom. It didn't help that Philip McDonald made me the lowest paid employee. I had spoken to Rosie Ivy upon starting but she in her wisdom ignored my request for a pay rise. It was a symptom of the stuttering mind that this occurred to me. Wendell Sugar managed to sort it out a few years later, but the damage to the stuttering self was done.

Just like walking, speaking is a subconscious process. I can remember how my 2 year old son started to walk. He was crawling for about 6 months, and then was using his hands to help himself stand up and finally using the wall for support, he stated to move around. He was programmed by the creator to do all these things. We, as parents, didn't tell him or show him anything. He is now communicating with words. He repeats the last word of any song we sing to him. That is his way of learning words. His mind is open to learning.

My friend, Alan Badminton from the United Kingdom, stuttered for over 50 years. Having been a policeman in the UK he used a device that stopped him from hearing is own voice for up to 12 hours a day, in order to do his job. He had failed at promotion board interviews due to the stuttering and after 20 years' service, he retired from the police force. I tried the same device when I was 19 years old. It made such a high pitched noise into my ear drums each time I spoke that I threw it out. Even though I stuttered like a parrot and my life at University was depressing I couldn't even use it for one day. It was awful. He shared this analogy with respect to stuttering treatment in one of his key note speeches delivered to the National Stuttering Association in the United States.

A man is walking along the road when he comes across another man on his hand and knees under a street lamp. Being a good samaritan, he stops and asks if he can be of help. "I am looking for my car keys", replies the man as he continues searching. The second man then joins him in the search. After about ten minutes, he asks, "Have you any idea of where you lost it?" "Yes", responds the first man, "over there, next to the trees." The second man asks, "Well, why are you looking here then?" "Because this is where the street light is" was his response.

This story is to show how the problem of stuttering has been tackled throughout the years. "Where the light is", meaning the mouth, jaw, throat area where the speech is produced is predominately the area of focus in stuttering treatment. This applies to nearly all forms of speech therapy. I believe stuttering is not only a speech problem, but a problem of the whole being.

"Our identity determines our thoughts that lead to our judgement, influence our actions and produce our results," says Mark Anastasi, New York Times best-selling author of The Laptop Millionaire. He adds, "It stands to reason that if one were to adopt the character traits, beliefs, values and identity of a wealthy, successful person, then they would also produce the same results as rich and successful people do!"

Successful people think differently, believe differently and behave differently to the rest of us. The unsuccessful people make the mistake of thinking it is only through education or luck that they achieved success and riches. What they don't realise is that it is their thought patterns and their subconscious beliefs that create their lives. These thoughts can be changed to make them successful. If the average person adopted the thinking patterns of the successful, then they would achieve the same results as them.

Therefore, in order for you to become free from the stuttering mindset, you need to eliminate this limiting belief and replace it with an empowering one, such as, "I speak with perfect control" or "I take my time when speaking."

Anastasi related the following in relation to people who want to become rich. As a person who had a stutter I reflected on these musings in relation to my speech and came up with three questions which everyone who stutters should ask, "Why do I stutter?", "Why do I feel the need to stutter?" and "How can I take full responsibility for what I have created in my life so far?"

These are very important questions because ultimately this is what everybody must do. Everybody ought to take full responsibility for what they have created and for what they have not yet created. If people do this then they will realise they have the power to create something new. If people say they want to be become free from stuttering, this really means that they want to create a new reality in their life – a reality which consists of them expressing themselves without doubt and fear. The way to achieve this is to start by taking back control of life and of the mind, which anyone can do by taking full responsibility for everything that their mind has produced – and has not yet produced – in their life so far. This is a scary thing to do. Most people would rather give up this responsibility by blaming others, and by being told what to do so that they can pass on the blame and complain to others if anything goes wrong.

Anastasi concludes, "Nothing will change in your life until you take back control of your creative power, until you realise your thinking has created your life exactly as it is today." It's about looking for silver linings, to coin a phrase, or putting your life carefully in perspective.

Are you afraid that one day you will wake up and not stutter? Does the excuse of having a stutter comfort you in the life you are leading? Can you imagine where you would be without a stutter? Now you don't have the excuse of the stutter, how is your life? Any different?

For the longest time I thought not stuttering would mean I would be happy. I thought I had found the Holy Grail when I attended a 3-day intensive course for stutterers. I even cried, when I got home after my first course, thinking about the wasted years. I did not stutter for the next three months, however nothing much changed in my life. I was still girlfriend less. I still didn't have any friends to hang out with on the weekends. Even though the stutter had all but gone during those three months I was no different. Like a bad penny the stutter returned much to my dismay.

It's only in living your life irrespective of the stutter, the stutter will cease to be a thorn in your life. If you are focused on removing the thorn, then the stutter will remain deeply ingrained.

Eric Edmeades in my book Rich Thinking says that what we believe is possible or not, determines the shape our lives take. "When somebody believes that all the opportunities are gone, they just see a lot of that evidence for all the opportunities being gone. When somebody believes that there is opportunity around every corner, then guess what they see around every corner? And so, I think that one of the things I have been working on since 1987 is constantly working to improve my own self-beliefs and my faith in the world, in the universe and life in general."

Elaborating on this further, Edmeades says: "I have this idea that beliefs are a little bit like a living organism: they need food, and the food of beliefs is evidence."

And the way in which a living organism keeps alive is by feeding. Edmeades says: "Belief is like a little living organism and it's going to look around for food, and so if somebody believes that there's no opportunity, they will read about other people's ideas and they will respond with a 'Oh, look. Another idea that's gone.' Or if somebody else has a really nice car, or is really successful, then, the negative person will say that all the opportunities are gone. And that negativity will get stronger and stronger. But I look at this the other way around," he says. "I want to feed the beliefs in the right way. I want to feed the positive beliefs. I believe there are opportunities around every corner, and you know what, I see them all the time. It doesn't mean I have to pursue them, but I see them. I see them for what they are and I am able to make a decision as to whether I want to chase down a given opportunity."

Beliefs affect every aspect of your life. They affect relationships, how you relate to your family and friends. They affect your money, how much you earn, spend and save. They affect your self-confidence, who you marry and even your personality: whether you are mostly happy or sad. Most people know that fear-based beliefs or emotions will hold you back from achieving your dreams. Even though, you are aware that you have limiting beliefs, life may not be what you want it to be. In order to make the kind of breakthrough, to live the extraordinary life you deserve, you will need to talk to your subconscious mind and transform your limiting beliefs.

A limiting belief is a thought that has evolved into a belief over time. A thought is just a thought. Every second, your brain generates countless thoughts. And each thought can be good or bad, empowering or disempowering.

A thought that is held long enough becomes a belief. Your thoughts or your mindset, which is your way of thinking, will help or hinder you. The key is to realise that your beliefs shape your reality. If you have a belief that no matter what, you will achieve success, then you will encounter coincidences in the universe which will aid you along the way, and your reality will manifest itself in front of your eyes. However, the contrary is also true.

Shelly Lefkoe, founder of Parenting the Lefkoe Way and cofounder and president of the Lefkoe Institute, an international self-improvement initiative, had an epiphany when she realised that so much of human suffering results from the beliefs that people hold about not being good enough or that they experience self-loathing due to things they perceive as having been mistakes or failures. She says these negative beliefs were at the root of so many problems such as: "Procrastination, depression, worrying about what people think, low self-esteem, fear of public speaking," and so on. In the broadest sense, Lefkoe has devoted herself to "helping people rid themselves of the beliefs that limit them from being free."

Consciously you want to speak like everyone. Can you honestly answer if there is any part of you that is happy that you stutter and are sitting on the sidelines of life?

ONE LAST THING

Thank you so much for reading the book. If you really enjoyed reading this, found it useful, interesting and inspiring I would be really grateful if you would post a review on Amazon.

Your support in writing a review will make a huge difference to me. I read all reviews personally and this will help me to improve my future work.

I really enjoyed writing this book and I am in the process of writing more books. You can email me at hellorama@thestutteringmind.com to be notified when I release a new book. This is not a newsletter sign up and you will not be sent unsolicited emails. To be perfectly honest I don't have the time. ☺ Your information will never be shared with anyone else.

Having read this book it is my wish that each and every one of you interacts with me and each other online to share what experiences, aha moments and insights you have all had. I look forward very much to connecting with all of you.

Things you can experience online:

An online video course that will guide you on your journey to freedom.

Audio MP3 of meditation and visualisation scripts.

Online community of readers where you can share your experiences.

Updates to the book, including future chapters and interviews.

FACEBOOK GROUP

J oin our Facebook group just for readers of The Stuttering Mind who want to be free from the shackles of stuttering. In this group we will be sharing insights, experiences, successes, strategies and tactics with each other so we can grow and support each other in our journey.

This is also a great supportive group for sharing and connecting with others who are on the journey to freedom.

https://www.facebook.com/groups/stutteringmind/

SOURCES

Day 72 - https://www.symmetrymagazine.org/article/the-particle-physics-of-you

Day 95 - www.lettersofnote.com/2011/11/delusion.html

Day 99 - http://www.nderf.org/Experiences/1anita_m_nde.html